THORA KRON, R.N., B.S.
Consultant in Team Nursing; formerly
Lecturer, Medical-Surgical Nursing
College of St. Scholastica
Duluth, Minnesota

The
Management
of
Patient Care

Putting Leadership Skills to Work

W. B. SAUNDERS COMPANY
Philadelphia · London · Toronto

W. B. Saunders Company: West Washington Square
Philadelphia, Pa. 19105

12 Dyott Street
London, WC1A   1DB

833 Oxford Street
Toronto 18, Ontario

The Management of Patient Care:
Putting Leadership Skills to Work — Third Edition   ISBN 0-7216-5527-0

Print No.:   9   8   7   6   5

4817 6

PREFACE

The material in this book is not entirely new. The reader will recognize much of it as coming from the two previous editions of *Nursing Team Leadership*. The author still believes that the philosophy and basic principles of team nursing provide a way for meeting the professional nursing responsibilities in the care of patients. The change in the title of the book reflects its increased coverage of management skills, not a reduction of the emphasis on leadership.

Many institutions are not giving their method of assignment a special name, partly because of the prejudice of the staff against the phrase, "team nursing," but mainly because they are trying new staffing patterns and feel that they do not fit into the pattern generally thought to be necessary for the practice of the team method of assignment. Team nursing cannot be reduced to a series of steps in a procedure telling the nursing practitioner exactly what to do and what not to do. Leadership in all aspects of patient care is still the responsibility of the professional nurse; however, sometimes nurses forget that philosophy and concepts may be implemented in a number of different ways to provide effective care for their patients.

This book is directed toward helping the professional nurse, especially the beginning practitioner, to understand the responsibilities in becoming a leader and to provide her with a simple guide to the various ways in which she may exercise leadership in the *Management of Patient Care*. The ideas and concepts presented in the book are only a starting point from which she can continue the study of methods of increasing her leadership skills in her own situation. Whatever her position – staff nurse, team leader, or head nurse – the professional nurse has the opportunity and the obligation to apply the principles of management in planning, directing, controlling, and evaluating the care of her patients.

The information about changes in nursing and nursing education has been brought up to date. Bibliographies have also been revised. New material has been added to explain in a simple way some of the methods that nurses can use to become more efficient in their arrangement of supplies and equipment, in studying and revising nursing techniques, in delegating job activities to the various workers on the nursing staff, and in the planning of their own activities. Additional information with illustrations has been included about the various approaches that may be used in the planning of nursing care and in the implementation of the care plan. The responsibility of the professional nurse to exercise her leadership through the management of patient care is emphasized throughout the book.

For those who want to continue the practice of team nursing, or to start this method of assignment of patient care, Part IV discusses the management of patient care using the principles of team nursing.

The phrase, "professional nurse," is employed throughout the book in the legal sense as used in licensure laws of each state except in some specific instances where the newer meaning of professional versus technical nursing is indicated.

The author wishes to thank the many professional nurses throughout the United States and Canada who have contributed so much by their many helpful suggestions and criticisms. Acknowledgment is extended to Helen Hill Blanz, LL.B., for her help in writing the section on the legal responsibilities in nursing.

Floodwood, Minnesota   THORA KRON

Beatitudes of a Leader

Blessed is the leader who has not sought the high places, but who has been drafted into service because of his ability and willingness to serve.

Blessed is the leader who knows where he is going, why he is going, and how to get there.

Blessed is the leader who knows no discouragement, who presents no alibi.

Blessed is the leader who knows how to lead without being dictatorial; true leaders are humble.

Blessed is the leader who seeks for the best for those he serves.

Blessed is the leader who leads for the good of the most concerned, and not for the personal gratification of his own ideas.

Blessed is the leader who develops leaders while leading.

Blessed is the leader who marches with the group, interprets correctly the signs on the pathway that leads to success.

Blessed is the leader who has his head in the clouds but his feet on the ground.

Blessed is the leader who considers leadership an opportunity for service.

Author Unknown

Reprinted from the *Blueprint Prepared for Local Leaders* by the National Education Association, Revised April, 1958.

CONTENTS

PART III.   PUTTING YOUR LEADERSHIP SKILLS
TO WORK

PART IV. PATIENT CARE MANAGEMENT AND
TEAM NURSING

PART ONE

LEADERSHIP — THE GREATEST CHALLENGE IN NURSING TODAY

For Yesterday is but a Dream,
And To-morrow is only a Vision;
But To-day well-lived makes every
  Yesterday a Dream of Happiness
And every To-morrow a Vision of Hope.
Look well therefore to this Day!

from The Salutation of the Dawn,
from the Sanskrit.

Chapter 1

A Look at Nursing Today

AIMS OF THE HOSPITAL

The primary aim of any hospital is to care for the sick. Additional aims, such as research and education, are formulated only because they will eventually lead either to the prevention of disease or to the improvement of patient care.

Each department within the hospital enlarges on this primary aim by relating its specific objectives and activities to the patient and his welfare. Thus, the dietary department is concerned with the nutritional care of the patient; the housekeeping department with the care of the patient's environment; the laboratory and x-ray departments with diagnostic and therapeutic techniques designed to help the patient in his recovery; and so on throughout every division within the hospital. In the nursing service department the aim becomes that of giving continuous good patient care to each individual.

NURSING—YESTERDAY AND TODAY

Changes in the Field of Medicine. The discovery of the principles of the microscope, the x-ray, photography, plastics, and the inventions of the twentieth century, such as the radio and television, and the use of the electron microscope and atomic energy have added impetus to medical research. These have brought about a rapid increase in the knowledge concerning the cause and treatment of many diseases.

New drugs are being used in the treatment of measles, smallpox, herpes simplex, influenza, and parkinsonism. Laser energy is being tried in the treatment of detached retina and certain malignant tumors. Scientists are giving the medical world additional information about the causes and treatment of certain heart, blood, and vascular diseases. The role of DNA in heredity is being studied. New and improved surgical techniques and instruments make possible, and even routine, some operations which a few years ago were unheard of. Hyperbaric surgery reduces mortality in operations on infants with congenital heart diseases. The use of intense cold in the treatment of certain conditions is being tried. Artificial hearts and lungs serve as temporary substitutes for those vital organs, and transplantation of organs such as kidneys, lungs, livers, spleens, and hearts are becoming almost commonplace, but with this increase in transplants have come some disturbing legal and ethical questions concerning who has title to a dead body and what death is. Electronic pacemakers keep damaged hearts beating rhythmically. In several instances severed limbs have been reattached successfully. Plastic materials and certain metals are being used to replace diseased sections of the body. Many facets of psychiatry, geriatrics, public health and sanitation are receiving attention of specialists in these fields.

Although great advances have been made, much remains to be done. At least 25 per cent of the population in the United States do not receive adequate medical care. The United States ranks 13th in infant mortality.* Life expectancy for United States males at age 45 is 27.0 years while men in 30 other countries have a longer life expectancy.** Health authorities are becoming increasingly concerned about pollution of our environment, the effects of the increasing noise level on people and property, and the illegal use of drugs by more people than ever before. Cancer and the common cold remain unconquered. Epidemics of infectious hepatitis, venereal disease, drug-resistant meningitis, and in 1968 a case of bubonic plague also point up the fact that we have not yet controlled communicable diseases. Continued advancement in space exploration necessitates research in space medicine.

The family doctor of yesteryear is almost unknown today, although recently the medical profession initiated action to bring him back as a "specialist in family medicine." The quantity and complexity of medical knowledge favor specialization and the increased use of consultation. Technicians, under the supervision of physicians who direct their work, are using the intricate equipment found in many areas of the modern hospital, for example, in the laboratory, the x-ray and the physical therapy departments.

Changes in Hospitals. Hospitals have also changed. At the beginning of the century a hospital was a big dismal building, thought

---

*"The Plight of the U.S. Patient." *Time,* Feb. 21, 1969, page 53.
**Reader's Digest Almanac and Yearbook.* Reader's Digest Association, Inc., Pleasantville, N.Y., 1969, page 335.

by many people to be a place of death. Now architecture and interior decoration are changing the physical appearance of the hospital while progress in medical science continues to eliminate the dangers that previously lurked within its walls. Gone are the high somber tan or dingy white walls and the narrow bare windows. The effect of color on the emotional response of the individual, and hence on his recovery, is now recognized; consequently, every effort is made to make the hospital bright and attractive as well as efficient and safe. Nursing stations are being planned so that the nurse can observe quickly and communicate easily with each patient.

Automation is becoming a part of hospital life. Intricate machines monitor the vital signs of patients, keeping minute by minute records of their progress. Automation can relieve nurses of up to 80 per cent of the paper work that now takes up most of their time. Some people foresee hospitals in which the patients' charts in their present form will be eliminated. Instead all information will be available through data processing by computers in the nursing stations. Data processing machines are now used in some hospitals to plan staffing, relay orders for laboratory and x-ray tests, supplies, and diets, transcribe doctors' orders, schedule patients' treatments, and chart nurses' notes.* These machines, in turn, have made necessary new knowledge and skills and additional personnel, usually ward clerks, to work with the machines. The use of disposable materials, including premixed infant formulas, medications, and equipment such as needles, syringes, and linen supplies, just to name a few, decreases the time needed to prepare and maintain these supplies as well as lessens the chance of infection.

In order to make more efficient use of personnel and equipment, some hospitals are grouping patients according to the care that they need. This system of progressive patient care includes an intensive care unit for the critically ill, a recovery room for patients immediately following surgery, regular care for the average patient, and minimal care or self-care units for convalescent patients and others who are ambulatory.

Changes in Social and Economic Conditions. With the decline in death rates has come a rise in the average age of the total population. Statisticians estimate that by 1970 the number of people 65 years and over will be at least 22 million, of whom approximately one-third will be over 75 years old.** These elderly people present special psychosocial and health care needs. In the meantime the total population continues to increase. This means that more and

---

*Given, C. W., and Given, Barbara: "Automation and Technology: A Key to Professionalized Care." *Nursing Forum* 8:1:74 (1969).
**Statistical Abstracts of the United States, 1962, 83rd annual edition, U.S. Bureau of the Census, Washington, D.C., 1962, U.S. Government Printing Office.

more people will need the services of doctors, nurses, hospitals, and nursing homes.

In addition to the increase in the number of people, several other factors are influencing the trend toward the greater use of medical and hospital facilities. The family is no longer a closely knit, stable, more or less independent entity. The shift is now away from the care of infirm, aged and ill persons by their own families. More and more the care of these individuals is assumed by service organizations such as nursing homes and hospitals. Doctors can no longer meet the demand for their services on a home-call basis, nor do they have available in their offices all the equipment and other facilities necessary for diagnostic and therapeutic care of their patients; therefore, they prescribe hospitalization.

The increased amount of information about health and disease, now being given in school and in popular literature, has made most people more health conscious. Along with this increased interest in health has come an increase in the number of subscriptions to the various hospitalization and health plans, thus increasing the demand for medical care and use of hospital facilities. However, the rise in the cost of living, including the cost of medical care and hospital facilities, has outrun the ability of many people to pay, especially those in the middle income range.* Throughout his book, *The Plot Against the Patient,* Fred Cook, Jr., seeks to prove that the problem of health is now "Big Business" with emphasis on profit rather than on the patient.**

Changes in Nursing and Nursing Education. In the past nurses did many of the housekeeping tasks around the hospital or home in addition to attending to the wants of their patients. Their duties were simple and entailed little knowledge or understanding of the patient's disease or the doctor's treatment. The nurse simply did as she was told. However, to keep pace with the changes in medicine, nurses have found it necessary to assume increasingly complex duties, to learn to work with new equipment safely and effectively and, consequently, to acquire more knowledge and understanding of medical diagnosis and treatment and of nursing itself. Various techniques, such as the administration of intravenous fluids, once thought to be within the realm of doctors only, are now being delegated to the professional nurse. As the care of the patient moved out of the home and into the hospital, the nursing profession found that it must supply more and more of that personal element hitherto provided by the patient's family.

The increase in the size and numbers of hospitals, the increased daily census of patients, the shortening of the work week, and the

---

*"The Plight of the U.S. Patient." *Time,* Feb. 21, 1969, pp. 53–54.
**Cook, Fred, Jr.: *The Plot Against the Patient.* Prentice-Hall, Inc., 1967.

growing number of complex skills and responsibilities have increased the demand for nurses beyond the available supply. New fields of endeavor, continually opening up to nurses in industry and public health, are taking some nurses who otherwise might be available for service in hospitals. An apparent decrease in the number of available professional nurses to care for patients has caused an increase in the use of practical nurses and ancillary personnel with more categories of workers being added every year.

Nursing education is confronted with the task of preparing the nurse to assume her role in society and in nursing. But what is that role? Several basic nursing programs are in existence—each with the expressed or implied objective of preparing nurses for first level positions, in other words, a staff nurse. But what do the phrases "first level" and "staff nurse" mean, especially since there is such a wide variation in the preparation of persons who are to fill this position? At the present time each employing agency defines what it expects of this person with the result that there is no standard job description of staff nurse responsibilities.

Members of the various health groups see the nurse in widely differing roles. Making a medical diagnosis and prescribing the treatment of the illness of a patient is the primary responsibility of the physician. Traditionally, the nurse has been considered one who "waits on" the doctor and performs the therapeutic techniques that he prescribes. On the other hand, hospital administrators think of the nurse as one who is capable of managing a section of the hospital, carrying out all administrative policies of the institution. In addition, the number of allied therapy personnel—laboratory and x-ray technicians, physical and occupational therapists, inhalation therapists, intravenous therapy teams, etc.—is increasing daily. The nurse is often responsible for coordinating the services of these people into the patient's schedule of care. As a result, she cannot find time to give nursing care to the patient. In other words, the nurse has allowed herself to become an assistant doctor, an assistant hospital administrator, a traffic manager, a service coordinator—a jack-of-all-trades but master of none. Although these duties are important to the patient's welfare, they do not constitute the giving of nursing care, which is the nurse's primary function. In her concern to perform these secondary duties, the nurse tends to neglect her main responsibility to the patient. In fact, she often delegates much of his care to ancillary workers.

Health agencies are trying different staffing categories and patterns. In place of the traditional head nurse, the ward or unit manager takes over the administrative duties usually assigned to the head nurse. This unit manager may be responsible to either the hospital administrator directly or to the director of nursing service. He may have one or more ward clerks or secretaries to do the more routine work of checking and ordering supplies, running errands, answering the telephone, and so forth. The head nurse is thus allowed to assume her professional responsibilities involving the care of her patients and supervision of her staff. Many hospitals have a general staffing secretary who plans the staffing hours for all nursing stations. In some instances the title of head nurse has been eliminated and she is now designated as coordinator of nursing care, thus emphasizing her responsibility for direct patient care rather than administration.* In other situations the head nurse functions as team leader, working directly with her staff in the planning and giving of patient care.

Because of the many changes occurring in nursing today and the resulting confusion in definition of roles and responsibilities, nurses and their professional organizations are trying to define and set up standards for nursing functions.

Bedside nursing has assumed the lowest status in nursing, and is usually assigned to practical nurses or aides. Yet what is the role of the professional nurse if not to give nursing care?

Marguerite Kakosh** says:

"Bedside care seems so much less important than the work of the head nurse or supervisor. 'I'm just a staff nurse' is the common remark. 'Today I was an aide. I did all the work that an aide does—gave baths, dressed and fed patients, assisted them into wheelchairs.' Was there really any difference in the practice of the aide and the nurse? Perhaps there is little reason to value it more highly. Until we are *able* and *enabled* to practice that quality of care that has inherent in it a growing source of satisfaction, we cannot expect respect for it. . . .

"Do we know *what* we are educating nurses for? Is my care the same as that given by the auxiliary? If there is no difference, then the *profession* of nursing will die and only the *occupation* of nursing will continue to exist!"

If nursing education is to meet its responsibility for preparing nursing practitioners able to give effective patient care, the educators must remember that there must be a common understanding and acceptance of the aims of nursing and of the various functions of nursing practitioners. At present there appears to be a wide gap in the goals of nursing education and the expectations of nursing service. This gap can be demonstrated in the difference between the stated aims of the various educational programs and the job descriptions of nursing service for levels of competency, especially of the new graduate. The kind of educational background is seldom considered either in job descriptions or in requirements for state licensure.

Because confusion exists concerning what nursing is and what nurses should do, discrepancies occur between what the nursing

---

*Hass, Ruth L.: "Our Nurses Are Nursing." *Minnesota Nursing Accent.* Minnesota Nurses Association, June, 1968, page 79.

**Kakosh, Marguerite: *Shortage: Nurses or Nursing?* Reprinted by permission from the *Canad. Nurse, 60*:131, (Feb., 1960).

student is taught and what she is expected to do as a graduate. As a student she is taught patient-centered care. Yet when she leaves the shelter of the nursing program, she may find that her work tends to become "procedure-centered" or "task-oriented" rather than "patient-centered." In small hospitals especially, she may find that she is expected to "take charge" of a nursing station because she is the only registered nurse available. Usually her education for a "first level" position has given her very little instruction or experience in administrative or supervisory activities.

The lack of understanding of common goals showed up in the emotional outburst that followed the suggestion for establishing different levels of nursing practice, namely, technical nursing and professional nursing.* At the insistence of nursing educators, nursing as a whole is moving slowly toward these two levels; however, there is still a feeling of resentment on the part of those nurses who do not yet understand the importance of the difference in the responsibilities of technical and professional nurse practitioners in planning and giving patient care.

Even now, without a formal division in levels of nursing practice, nurses are not always sure what their responsibilities do include; therefore they judge their work on the basis of techniques alone, rather than on how well they are identifying and meeting the needs of their patients. In view of some of the criticism of hospitals and nurses, the nursing profession appears to be failing to give what the public considers good care. Studies seem to indicate that a patient is most concerned with his physical comfort, with being told what to expect, and with having his questions answered. In other words, nurses are most often criticized for their lack of communication and consideration of the personal needs of the patient. On the other hand, these same studies indicated that nurses felt that giving treatments and medications on time and maintaining a safe environment were the most important aspects of the patients' care.**

Part of the responsibility of nursing education in both the technical and professional nursing programs is to help the nursing student learn how to function in a situation which is less than ideal, to determine priorities both in nursing activities and in meeting patient problems, and to use herself most effectively. More than anything else the nursing instructor must encourage students to continue to accept and try new ideas and methods in order to improve their nursing practice. At the same time the instructor should prepare the student to overcome some of the frustrations occurring

---

*American Nurses' Association. "Position on Education for Nursing." *Am. J. Nursing.* 65:12:106 (Dec., 1965).

**Abdellah, Fay G., and Levine, Eugene. "Developing a Measure of Patient and Personnel Satisfaction with Nursing Care." *Nursing Research,* 5:2:100 (Feb., 1957).

with progress by helping her realize that change occurs slowly because people resist change when they feel it constitutes a threat to their security, economic or emotional or both. Frustration caused by discrepancies between expectations acquired during education and conditions encountered in meeting job requirements may be a contributing factor in causing a number of nurses to become inactive shortly after graduation.

A suggestion advanced recently by some people has to do with the setting up of career ladders. In its simplest form the ladder allows the registered nurse without a degree to take additional work in order to obtain a baccalaureate degree. Some programs are now in existence that allow the licensed practical nurse to receive credit for her vocational program to enable her, with a short period of additional education, to be qualified to take the examinations to become a registered nurse. Other proponents start with the nursing aide and continue upward, placing the surgeon at the apex. To ascend this ladder a worker can receive "credits" for job experience and on-the-job training, as well as formal educational courses. Several problems arise from this idea. First, the question arises about which health workers can be allowed to climb such a ladder. Second, some of those in favor of such a ladder tend to visualize nursing as a series of manual tasks of varying complexity so that the worker could move upward by simply learning a few more skills. They do not recognize the need for acquiring new attitudes and goals and how difficult this may be because of previous education and experience. Third, there is the question of evaluating the many different kinds of job experiences and training and deciding how much "credit" would be allowed.

In addition many proponents of the career ladder suggest bringing in more unskilled persons who, after their on-the-job training, would work as nursing aids. This would allow more experienced workers time to receive the training necessary to move up to the next level.* Some suggest this system as a means of combating poverty with the introduction of additional worker categories and emphasize worker satisfaction,** but show little if any concern for the recipient of the worker's ministrations—that is, the patient. The introduction of additional categories of workers can lead only to further fragmentation of care of the patient who is already confused by the large number of personnel with whom he must deal. Another suggestion, first proposed by Duff and Hollingshead*** and now espoused by the American Medical Association,**** is that nurses should function as

---

*"Ladder System Outlined, Aide to R.N." *Am. J. Nursing*, 68:8:1743 (Aug., 1968).

**Riessman, Frank: *Strategies Against Poverty*. Random House, 1969, pp. 22, 27.

***Duff, Raymond S., and Hollingshead, August B.: *Sickness and Society*. Harper and Row, 1968, p. 384.

****"AMA Unveils Surprise Plan to Convert RN into Medic." *Am. J. Nursing*, 70: 4:691 (April, 1970).

physicians' assistants and be responsible for the medical care on the patient unit under the direction of the physician, and that medical auxiliaries replace nurses and be given the opportunity to advance in a career of medical care. Note the omission, or perhaps intentional elimination, of the word, *nursing*.

In practice many registered nurses are already functioning in this capacity, since they are concerned with giving medications, starting intravenous infusions, diagnosing cardiac arrest and prescribing appropriate measures of treatment, and working with monitoring machines and other intricate equipment and techniques while the L.P.N. and nursing assistant give the "nursing" care at the bedside. It is ironic that the registered nurse is so ready to give away her right to be an independent professional practitioner in planning and giving nursing care and chooses instead the non-professional, secondary role of a physician's assistant.

WORDS AND CONCEPTS USED IN NURSING TODAY

Since we use many words and phrases to describe our nursing philosophy, aims, and functions, perhaps we should consider some of them briefly at this time. As always, assignment of meanings to words is not easy, for each person tends to superimpose his own meaning over dictionary definitions. Furthermore, some words may be used in a number of ways and consequently have a variety of meanings.

Need.   One of the most frequently used words is *need*. We have a number of ways of classifying needs — basic or physiologic, supportive, emotional, economic, and so on. A *need* may be defined as that which the individual must have in order to survive or function within limits which society, including medicine, considers normal. Oxygen, water, food, and elimination of wastes are absolutely necessary for survival. Other needs that influence the person's ability to function include physical comfort, sexual satisfaction, mental as well as physical activity and rest, along with knowing what is happening, being accepted by other people, feeling worth something to others.

Problem.   As we use this word in our everyday living, it usually means anything that we do not know how to manipulate or cope with. However, in nursing it has a different meaning. A *problem* is the result of an unmet need to which the patient responds in a variety of ways that we call symptoms, emotional or physical, verbal or non-verbal. An unmet need may already be present, or the nurse may foresee a future need and meet it by appropriate nursing measures, thereby preventing the occurrence of a problem. Therefore, a nursing problem is a condition with which the nurse can help her patient by meeting the underlying need or helping the patient to meet his own need.

Abdellah classifies nursing problems as *overt* and *covert*.* An *overt nursing problem* is one which is discernible to the nurse and perhaps to the patient and his family. A *covert nursing problem* is one not readily discernible. The covert problem may cause unrelated overt behavior, e.g., constantly putting on the call light and asking for "little" things to be done. The nurse must determine the real reason for the patient's putting on his call light if she is to identify the covert problem correctly and determine an effective way to meet the need which is the primary cause of this behavior. On the other hand, the patient's physical symptoms may cause problems, overt or covert.

A patient was unable to move his arms. This was a physical symptom due to the effects of his disease condition. A nursing student, while caring for him, readily recognized the effect this symptom would have on the patient's ability to feed himself or to get a drink of water. With a little help she also realized that the patient might be embarrassed by having to ask for help when using the bedpan or urinal and consequently might not ask for them when he should. The failure to meet elimination needs could lead to bladder infection and constipation. In this instance the nurse, by recognizing the symptom —inability to move his arms—could foresee possible nursing problems and, with appropriate planning, prevent their occurrence.

The patient and the nurse do not always identify the same conditions as being problems. For this reason those which interest the patient or are the cause of his symptoms, whether he recognizes them or not, I prefer to call *patient problems.* The responsibility of the nurse almost always is to start with what the patient considers important because, unless she is able to help him with that, he may refuse help in those areas which she has identified as nursing problems. For example, hygienic care of the skin and change of position are ways of preventing skin breakdown or promoting healing when breakdown does occur. However, the patient may refuse to turn. The nurse may turn the patient as often as she decides is necessary and may prevent any skin breakdown. However, if she fails to recognize the refusal to turn as a symptom of an unmet need or patient problem (covert nursing problem, if you prefer) and consequently does not determine the cause of this behavior, she will be unable to meet her patient's needs in this area. If turning the patient is all that she does, and she does not meet the underlying need, she is giving procedure-centered care rather than professional nursing care.

Nursing Process.   Problem-solving techniques are employed in identifying nursing and patient problems and in planning and giving nursing care. The use of these techniques is now being called the *nursing process* and involves the nurse, the patient, and his family.

---

*Abdellah, Fay G. et al.: *Patient-Centered Approaches to Nursing.* Macmillan Co., 1960, pp. 6–7.

COLLECTION OF INFORMATION ABOUT THE PATIENT. We can get information from the doctor or other members of the health team, from the patient's chart, from his family, and from literature which discusses how the disease affects a person. However, the best source of information is the patient himself. Here we need to use our various senses—smell, touch, and sight as well as hearing. Communication with the patient is important, both verbal and nonverbal. We must perceive the whole person and recognize those interrelated activities which influence his behavior. In collecting our information we must avoid preconceived ideas or assumptions which may result in incorrect perception of the patient as a person and of his needs. We must be able to recognize the effects that illness, culture, social environment, age, sex, and other factors have on the patient. In other words, we must get to know the patient and try to understand him in order to identify his needs.

NURSING ASSESSMENT. This involves an interpretation of accumulated data. Interpretation, however, is based upon knowledge which is understood and therefore can be related to the patient in a personal way. Assessment includes, in addition to the ability to see meaningful relationships, the ability to use one's judgment and make decisions about nursing problems. This identification of nursing problems is sometimes called making a *nursing diagnosis.*

PLANNING NURSING INTERVENTION. Other phrases applied to this technique include planning *nursing therapy, nursing action,* and *nursing care.* Based upon her perception of patient needs combined with her knowledge of the biological, behavioral, medical, and nursing sciences, the nurse determines not only *what* to do but *how* to do it. At the same time she determines priorities of nursing activities and decides upon the sequence of these activities and who will perform them.

IMPLEMENTING THE NURSING CARE PLAN. The plan of care is of no value to the patient unless it is put into action; therefore the nurse is responsible for guiding and helping those who work with the patient. The management of patient care involves a knowledge of administrative principles and supervisory techniques and an understanding of how to meet the needs of the patient. The nurse's responsibility for effective management in the care of her patients is the main theme of this book.

EVALUATION. The nursing process must include evaluation, both during administration of care and upon its completion. In order to make a valid evaluation the nurse must have set up expected goals and criteria of performance. She should evaluate each of the steps in the process as well as the final product, i.e., the care of the patient and his response. Here the patient, his family, and other members of the health team can participate.

Total Patient Care. Total patient care or comprehensive care is usually defined as meeting all the needs of the patient—emotional, spiritual, physical, environmental, social, economic, and rehabilitative, including all teaching needed in any of these areas. Total care recognizes the patient as a member of a family and a community and strives to help both the patient and his family make the necessary adjustments to his limitations. The nurse recognizes that many people will contribute to the total care of her patient but that she may need to act as coordinator to some who render services to her patient.

When the nurse cares for a patient with congestive heart failure, she reviews all she knows about the normal functioning of the heart and circulation and the possible effects that this malfunctioning may have on the various life processes of a person. She knows that the patient needs rest—physical and mental. His drugs, treatments, food, and nursing care, as well as his environment and rehabilitation must be planned with this need in mind. He must be taught which activities, foods, and drugs are good for him and why. He must also learn which ones are contraindicated so that he will understand and derive the most benefit from his hospital care. He must realize the effect that emotions may have on his condition, and he must understand what to do about his job, and his place in his family and community. This is total patient care.

Individualized Patient Care. This is sometimes called *patient-centered care*. Is it the same as total care? Yes, except that it goes a step further. It involves understanding the background knowledge necessary in total patient care but it also includes a knowledge and understanding of the patient as an individual and of his specific needs. The nurse's knowledge and understanding serve as the basis for selection of principles and appropriate nursing measures to solve nursing problems peculiar to this patient.

Good Nursing Care. Another phrase which has different meanings to different people is *nursing care*. To some, nursing care still means only the performance of procedures according to predetermined steps or established hospital policies. Frances Reiter Kreuter, in her discussion of nursing care,* insists that the administration of medicines, tests, and treatments is a nursing *operation* which cannot be called nursing *care* unless the nurse helps the patient during the experience. In other words, nursing procedures and duties are not the same as nursing care. One of the simplest, yet most inclusive, definitions of nursing is given by Virginia Henderson: ". . . to assist the individual, sick or well, in the performance of those activities contributing to health or its recovery (or to peaceful death) that he would perform unaided if he had the necessary strength, will or knowledge. And to do this in such a way as to help him gain inde-

---

*Kreuter, Frances Reiter. "What is Good Nursing Care?" *Nurs. Outlook.* May, 1957, pp. 302–304.

pendence as rapidly as possible."* This means not only performing those duties delegated by the medical profession and by hospital administration but also helping the patient physically, emotionally, and spiritually.

This brief discussion previews the ideas, principles, and techniques which will be explored throughout this book.

STUDY QUESTIONS

1. What do you think is the main contribution of the nurse to the doctor-nurse-patient relationship? Why?

2. What do you think is the most important contribution the nurse can make to the patient? Why?

3. How would you answer when someone says, "I didn't see a nurse during the entire week I was in the hospital"?

4. What do *you* mean when you say someone is a *good* patient? Analyze your meaning.

5. What do you mean when you describe someone as being a *good* nurse?

6. List as many changes as you can that have occurred in the field of medicine in your own hospital in the last five years. What brought about each change? What were the effects of each change on the duties and responsibilities of the professional nurse?

7. Discuss what you think are the major problems confronting nurses today.

8. Formulate your own definition for the following:
   a. Patient problem
   b. Nursing problem
   c. Nursing diagnosis
   d. Nursing intervention
   e. Nursing care
   f. Priorities of nursing care

9. It is possible to perform a procedure and not give nursing care? Why?

---

*Henderson, Virginia. "The Nature of Nursing." *Am. J. Nursing*, 64:8:63 (Aug., 1964).

Chapter 2

Responsibilities of the Professional Nurse in the Management of Patient Care

As stated in the Preface, the phrase professional nurse is used throughout most of this book in the legal sense as in the licensure laws of each state. The reader should understand that each nurse has varying capabilities because of her inherent abilities and her educational and experiential background; consequently the philosophy and skills displayed by one nurse in the performance of her nursing responsibilities will be different from those of another nurse.

VARIOUS ASPECTS OF PATIENT CARE

The professional nurse is responsible for the care her patients receive. The amount of responsibility she must assume will be determined by her job and her assignment within the employing agency. The head nurse is responsible for all care given by her staff to the patients on her station. A staff nurse or team leader may be responsible for the care of a smaller number of patients, depending on the methods of assignment used on the unit. This does not mean that the professional nurse can or should give all the care needed by her patients. The use of L.P.N.'s, nursing assistants and orderlies is necessary, and the professional nurse is responsible for using these people effectively and for helping and supervising them. This means she must know what activities and responsibilities she can delegate to each person and how to ensure an adequate performance of these assigned duties.

TABLE 1. Nursing Responsibilities for Patient Care

| Dependent Functions — Delegated | | Independent Functions — Professional |
Administrative	Medical	Professional Nursing
Agency policies Agency procedures	Delegated medical therapy based upon the medical diagnosis and plan of medical therapy.	Make a nursing diagnosis based upon assessment of the patient. Plan nursing intervention (nursing care) based upon the nursing diagnosis and aim of nursing therapy.
Coordinating agency services to aid in the diagnosis, therapy, rehabilitation, etc. of the patient based upon policy, procedure, and orders given by the doctor.		The professional nurse may delegate nursing care to L.P.N.'s and nursing aides, but there are some responsibilities that she cannot delegate:
The professional nurse may delegate many of these activities to other personnel (housekeeping, dietary, and laboratory departments, ward secretary, and others) and to L.P.N.'s and nursing assistants.		Assessment of the patient Making a nursing diagnosis Planning nursing therapy Evaluating patient care Supervising and helping those who give delegated care to patients.
The activities necessary in the execution of these functions are usually found on the treatment and medication card (Medical Care Plan) in the Kardex.		The activities necessary in the performance of professional nursing functions are found on the nursing order card (Nursing Care Plan) usually in the Kardex.

Although the professional nurse is responsible for patient care, there are many aspects of that care (see Table 1). These include the dependent functions delegated by the employing agency and the patient's physician, and those functions related to the planning and giving of nursing care which are the professional nurse's primary responsibility as an independent practitioner.

Dependent Functions. The nursing staff must follow the employing agency's policies and procedures. These are set up to facilitate good general care of a patient, and to prevent wasted time and effort and excessive use of supplies by the staff. Because they are dictated by administration, they are dependent responsibilities. But strict adherence to a policy or a procedure does not always insure the best, or even safe, care for the patient. A policy may state that each patient should have a daily bath. However, such a procedure could be dangerous for a patient acutely ill following a myocardial infarction. Someone must interpret the policy according to the needs of the patient. This is the responsibility of the professional nurse in exercising her function as an independent practitioner.

The physician brings his patient to the hospital and gives the staff directions about the care he wants his patient to receive. This care is also a dependent function because the staff depends upon the orders left by the doctor. The execution of such orders usually involves following a policy or performing a procedure previously accepted by the hospital. Furthermore, the doctor's orders depend upon his medical diagnosis and are related to relief of symptoms or cure of a disease and not necessarily to helping the patient through the experience, i.e., they do not constitute nursing care even though they are given by the nursing staff.

Independent Functions. The physician's orders may be modified or interpreted by the nurse through her right to use her professional knowledge and judgment. The doctor says to give Demerol 75 to 100 mg. p.r.n. for discomfort. The nurse must determine whether or not the patient needs Demerol and if so, how much. Perhaps the doctor says to force fluids to 2000 cc. and make up any deficit with intravenous fluids. The nurse, acting as a professional practitioner, determines what fluids the patient prefers and can have, and then she plans a schedule so that the intake is adequately spaced throughout the day. Thus she helps her patient avoid the many dangers that attend the intravenous administration of fluids.

The nurse may delegate to other members of the nursing staff some aspects of nursing care after she has planned what the patient needs and how the care should be given. Here again, she is guided by policy as well as by her assessment of the patient's needs. Job descriptions indicate which activities she may assign to the L.P.N. and which to the nursing assistant or orderly; however, she must evaluate the worker's ability to perform a particular technique. Policy may allow an aide to help a patient get up into a chair, but if the patient needs special help when getting up, the nurse must decide whether the aide can meet these special needs, or whether someone with more knowledge should be assigned to help the patient.

The primary function of the professional nurse is to use the nursing process. As previously described, this includes the collection of information and the assessment of the patient, leading to the making of a nursing diagnosis. Then she must plan the care of her patient and put her plan into action by delegating activities and supervising and teaching those who give the care. She may delegate many procedures and duties to auxiliary personnel; however, she cannot delegate her professional responsibility for planning, supervising, and evaluating the care that the nursing staff gives to the patients. Finally, she must evaluate the effectiveness of her planned nursing therapy.

WHAT INFLUENCES THE ROLE OF THE NURSE

Every person fills many roles in today's society, which defines each role according to its expectations of behavior. The doctor expects a certain pattern of behavior for a nurse. Very often he does not differentiate among the levels of practice present in nursing today. The hospital administrator sees the nurse in a very different role. The patients and their families have other expectations, depending upon their culture, past experiences, and the degree of illness of the patient.

The nurse may visualize herself in still another role, which is determined by her personal philosophy about nursing and about herself as a person. Other factors that influence her are her educational background, the amount of active nursing experience she has had, and her desire and ability to accept leadership responsibilities.

If she sees herself as responsible only for ordered procedures and care, she will plan her patient's care so that it is task-oriented, emphasizing procedures. If she is unwilling to accept responsibility for directing and supervising other members of the nursing staff, she will certainly be unhappy in any position requiring leadership and will probably prefer the functional method of assignment. If, however, she is interested in patients, their needs, and how to help people, her care will be more patient-centered even when she is performing techniques. This behavior will show up whether she has had a technical or a professional nursing education.

If the nurse is willing to accept the responsibility which goes with using her judgment and making decisions necessary in the practice of the independent functions in nursing, her practice will demonstrate her philosophy. The more knowledge, understanding, and experience she has the better she will be able to fill the role of a leader in the management of nursing care.

VARIOUS METHODS USED IN THE ASSIGNMENT OF THE CARE OF PATIENTS

Functional Assignment. This method emphasizes the dependent functions of nursing responsibility and the assignment of procedures and duties usually found on the treatment and medication part of the Kardex. In other words, the nurses' aides give baths, feed patients, and take T.P.R.'s while the registered nurse is assigned as the "medication nurse." The head nurse is responsible for the direction and supervision of her entire staff, with each person directly responsible to her. Any questions and reports are directed toward the head nurse, and little communication takes place among the staff about patient care. The "medication nurse" does not have the authority or the opportunity to supervise the care given by other members on the staff. If the L.P.N. is assigned to this activity, she cannot supervise the nursing staff as they give patient care. When the nurse is giving medications, she seldom has much time to spend with patients, talking with them or observing their response to their medications or to their care.

In functional assignments there is little or no coordination among the fragments of patient care. Frequently the patient must repeat requests or questions to each worker who enters his room. Is it any wonder that he begins to doubt that anyone knows about his care or considers him as a person?

The head nurse who is more concerned with patients as individuals will try to pass on directions and information that will tend to make the care somewhat more individualized. However, directions and information are usually given verbally and may therefore be forgotten. Furthermore, they may not reach every worker who is to care for the patient. When using the functional method of assignment, the head nurse seldom has time to help her staff learn the best way to meet the patient's needs or to evaluate their conditions and care, so only the more obvious needs may be taken care of.

Emphasis is usually on "get the work done," and the worker judges her performance by how many baths she gave, or beds she made, or medications she administered.

Team Assignment. In this method some decentralization of responsibility occurs because the head nurse delegates some of her activities to the registered nurse on the nursing staff. This person is usually called the team leader, and is responsible for making assignments and directing and supervising other staff personnel, called team members, as they give patient care. The team members may be registered nurses, L.P.N.'s, nurses' aides, and orderlies. The team method, when it is used according to its original philosophy, emphasizes the entire team's knowing about the patient and his needs and working together to give patient-centered care. The team members are encouraged to go to their team leader with questions and observations about their patients. This method utilizes leadership by a registered nurse in planning nursing to meet the needs of the patient and insuring continuity of nursing care by means of the written nursing care plan. The team leader, rather than the head nurse, directs and supervises her team members. Without these basic essentials, care usually reverts to the old functional method of assignment, regardless of the name given to it.

LEGAL ASPECTS OF NURSING PRACTICE

It is almost impossible to give specific information about the legal aspects inherent in the practice of nursing. Although every state has a nursing practice law, each state sets its own standards and often does not define, except in general terms, what constitutes the practice of professional and technical nursing or of practical nursing. Consequently, the interpretation and practice of nursing functions and responsibilities and the standards of care may vary from area to area within a state as well as throughout the nation.

Every nurse, is, first of all, a citizen and, as a citizen, must be willing to assume the responsibilities imposed by law. Although nursing practice laws do benefit the nurse, they are mainly concerned with the protection of people. In nursing, as in few other professions, the practitioner is directly responsible for the safety and welfare of people; therefore, the nurse must be well informed about the ways of meeting her legal obligations in the practice of her profession within her own state and community.

According to Lesnik and Anderson, seven areas have been legally identified as professional nursing activities. In the area involving the execution of the physician's orders the nurse's activities may be considered to be dependent; however, in the other areas she is an independent practitioner. Today the registered nurse is finding that one of her major responsibilities is the direction and supervision of the allied health personnel who give patient care; therefore, she must recognize that she may be liable if her actions result in another person acting in a negligent manner. The professional nurse may be liable not only for the injurious acts of her agents, e.g., the practical nurse, done within the scope of authority but also for her failure to carry out her legal responsibility of directing and supervising the care of the patient, including that given by licensed practical nurses and other auxiliary personnel.

Legal Responsibility for Planning the Nursing Care of the Patient. As has been stated several times previously and certainly implied by Lesnik and Anderson, the professional nurse must give care which goes beyond mere execution of the doctor's orders or adherence to hospital policy. In this area she has the duty to render that quality and quantity of care as given by the average nurse in the community at that time. This care must be planned and is based upon the nurse's application of principles found in the biologic, the physical and the social sciences.

This plan of care necessitates the assessment of the patient's nursing needs, the making of a nursing diagnosis, the determination of appropriate nursing measures, and the execution of the plan in order to achieve the aim of nursing care.

All of these are professional nursing activities and are necessary in the management of patient care. The nurse may plan the care of her patient by herself, or she may encourage other members of the staff to contribute. When put into written form, the care plan provides the staff with a constant reminder and guide about what they hope to accomplish for the patient. It also provides the professional nurse with a basis for evaluating both the care of the patient and the work of each staff member.

Legal Implications Related to the Assignment of Patient Care.
Since a registered nurse usually works with one or more auxiliary
persons, she must realize that some legal responsibility is present.
Concern for the safety and well-being of the patient is of primary
importance when assignments are made. Job titles such as nurses'
aide, or even licensed practical nurse, do not indicate the degree of
skill or understanding of the individual. Failure of the registered
nurse to recognize this may make her liable for injury caused by an
act of one of her subordinates. She must consider the needs of the
patient, the capabilities of her staff, and the policies of the organization when making assignments to perform nursing techniques or to
execute any therapeutic treatments which she may delegate to other
personnel.

An important aspect in making assignments involves the manner in which they are given. Each person must understand exactly
what she is to do, thus defining the scope of authority of the subordinates or agents and, consequently, limiting the liability of the
professional nurse. Errors in giving treatments or doing any part of
the patient's care may occur when directions do not indicate clearly
who is to perform the care or what and how it is to be done. Every
worker should receive a complete report about her patients and an
explanation of her assignment before beginning her day's work.

Legal Responsibility to Provide Supervision.   Negligence may
result from acts of omission as well as acts of commission. The law
defines *direction* broadly as governing, ruling, or ordering and *supervision* as overseeing or inspecting. Gradually, nursing is accepting a
broader definition of supervision, perhaps implied in the term *overseeing,* to include teaching and guidance of the worker to help him to
do his best. This broader definition implies that a qualified person
observes the worker and helps and teaches him whenever the need is
observed. The responsibility related to assignment of patient care is
not discharged until the care is completed in the way the registered
nurse desires. To insure completion of all assignments she must
supervise each worker during as well as after the giving of patient
care.

**Legal Responsibility Involving Observing and Reporting Re-
sponses of the Patient and Evaluating Nursing Care.**   Here the
nurse has a professional and legal obligation to use all information
obtained by her staff. One of the major differences between the
professional nurse and the allied nursing personnel is the ability and
obligation of the professional nurse to interpret and evaluate facts
and decide upon the appropriate action.

The nurse must demand and get all the information she can
about each patient; therefore, she must help other nursing personnel to learn what to observe and must impress upon them the
importance of reporting their observations and findings to her. She

may wish to verify these observations before taking final action, but she is legally responsible for her use of all the information that is brought to her attention. Obtaining and using such information, whether to help in planning the care of a patient or in evaluating the care already given, is an important part of the registered nurse's responsibility for supervision.

No specific criteria can be set down by which negligence may be determined. In general, negligence may be shown if the nurse fails to exercise due care or demonstrates lack of reasonable skill in her performance compared to that expected of a nurse with similar education and experiences in that community at the time of the specific incident.

The professional nurse must keep informed about hospital policies, including job descriptions for herself and her staff. There is always an element of danger when someone says, "We always do it this way." All policies and job descriptions should be in writing and kept up-to-date so that there is never any question concerning what should and should not be done, thus helping to protect both the employing agency and the employee.

Each individual is held liable for her own acts, whether she is a registered nurse, a licensed practical nurse, a nursing student, or a nurses' aide. The professional nurse, however, has a moral obligation, although not a legal one, to help each worker to understand her legal obligations toward the patient.

Other people will learn by watching the professional nurse; therefore, she must be careful that she always demonstrates high standards of nursing practice, ethically as well as legally. She should help her staff to understand their legal obligations involving making medical diagnoses, offering opinions about treatment, slander, and invasion of privacy, especially concerning confidential information. In these areas the nurse can teach both by her actions and by giving specific information.

STUDY QUESTIONS

1. What is the difference between patient care and nursing care (nursing intervention)?

2. What are the main areas found in patient care for which the nursing staff is responsible?

3. Discuss how the responsibilities of the head nurse differ from those of the staff nurse for patient care. For nursing care?

4. Give some examples of duties which the registered nurse can delegate to an L.P.N. in your hospital. To a nurses' aide? To an orderly? What cannot be delegated? Why? Are you including only techniques (procedures) among those responsibilities that cannot be delegated? Why?

5. What are the various roles you must fill in your everyday life and in your nursing position?

6. What is the difference between the functional method of assignment of patient care and the team method? What are the essential activities which differentiate the functional from the team method? How are the legal responsibilities of the registered nurse affected in team nursing?

7. According to the legal definition of the functions of a practical nurse, why cannot the L.P.N. function as a team leader? (Note the word is *function*, not *be assigned*.) Remember that the team leader must be someone who is qualified to take the responsibility for planning and directing patient care and supervising those who give the care.

PART ONE BIBLIOGRAPHY

Books

Abdellah, Fay G., et al.: *Patient-Centered Approaches to Nursing*. The Macmillan Company, New York, 1960.
Cook, Fred, Jr.: *The Plot Against the Patient*. Prentice-Hall, Inc., Englewood Cliffs, N.J., 1967.
Duff, Raymond S., and Hollingshead, August B.: *Sickness and Society*. Harper & Row Publishers, Inc., New York, 1968. Chapts. 5, 7, 11, and 13.

Pamphlets and Journals

AMA Unveils Surprise Plan to Convert R.N. into Medic. Am. J. Nursing, 70:4:691, April, 1970.
And Now Practical Doctors? (Editorial) Am. J. Nursing, 67:7:1415, July, 1967.
Aydelotte, Myrtle K.: *Issues of Professional Nursing: The Need for Clinical Excellence.* Nursing Forum, 7:1:73, 1968.
Bennett, Leland R.: *. . . That Nurses May Become Extinct.* Nurs. Outlook, 18:1:28, Jan., 1970.
Benz, Edward G.: *Nursing Service.* Hospitals, 43:7:157, April 1, 1969.
Cherescavish, Gertrude: *The Expanding Role of the Professional Nurse in a Hospital.* Nursing Forum, 3:4:9, 1964.
Conant, Lucy H.: *Closing the Practice-Theory Gap.* Nurs. Outlook, 15:11:37, Nov., 1967.
Couter, Pearl Parvin: *Programing for Nursing Service.* Nurs. Outlook, 15:9:33, Sept., 1967.
Fenninger, Leonard D.: *Education in the Health Professions.* Nurs. Outlook, 16:4:30, April, 1968.
Feuer, Helen Denny: *Operation Salvage.* Nurs. Outlook, 15:11:54, Nov., 1967.
Ginzberg, Eli: *Nursing and Manpower Realities.* Nurs. Outlook, 15:11:26, Nov., 1967.
Given, C. W., and Given, Barbara: *Automation and Technology: A Key to Professionalized Care.* Nursing Forum, 8:1:74, 1969.
Greenough, Katharine: *Determining Standards for Nursing Care.* Am. J. Nursing, 68:10:2153, Oct., 1968.
Hall, Lydia E.: *Nursing—What Is It?* Canadian Nurse, 60:2:150, Feb., 1964.
Hass, Ruth L.: *Our Nurses Are Nursing.* Minnesota Nursing Accent, Minnesota Nurses Ass'n, June, 1968, pg. 79.
Health Care Needs—Basis for Change. National League for Nursing, No. 20-1332, 1968.
Henderson, Virginia: *The Nature of Nursing.* Am. J. Nursing, 64:8:63, Aug., 1964.
Johnson, Dorothy E.: *A Philosophy of Nursing.* Nurs. Outlook, 7:4:198, April, 1959.
Johnson, Dorothy E.: *Significance of Nursing Care.* Am. J. Nursing, 61:11:63, Nov., 1961.
Kakosh, Marguerite: *Shortages: Nurses or Nursing?* Canadian Nurse, 60:2:131, Feb., 1960.
Kreuter, Frances R.: *What Is Good Nursing Care?* Nurs., Outlook, 5:5:302, May, 1957.
Kriegel, Julia: *Are We Earning Our Salaries?* Nurs. Outlook, 15:12:60, Dec., 1967.

Ladder System Outlined, Aide to R.N. Am. J. Nursing, *68*:8:1743, Aug., 1968.

Levine, Eugene: *Nurse Manpower—Yesterday, Today, and Tomorrow.* Am. J. Nursing, *69*:2:290, Feb., 1969.

Lindsey, Margaret: *Professional Standards—Whose Responsibility?* Am. J. Nursing, *62*:11:84, Nov., 1962.

Mercadante, Lucille R.: *Unit Manager Plan Gives Nurses More Time to Care for the Patients.* Modern Hospital, *99*:2:73, Aug., 1962.

Nahm, Helen: *Nursing Dimensions and Realities.* Am. J. Nursing, *65*:6:96, June, 1965.

National Commission for the Study of Nursing and Nursing Education. Am. J. Nursing, *70*:2:279, Feb., 1970.

Neighbor, Howard D.: . . . *About Nursing Education.* Nurs. Outlook, *18*:3:34, March, 1970.

New, Peter Kong-Ming: *Another Approach to Professionalism.* Am. J. Nursing, *65*:2:124, Feb., 1965.

Nurses, Nursing, and the AMA. Am. J. Nursing, *70*:4:808, April, 1970.

Perspectives for Nursing. National League for Nursing. No. 11-1166, 1965.

Price, Elmina: *Data Processing: Present and Potential.* Am. J. Nursing, *67*:12:2558, Dec., 1967.

Ramphal, Marjorie: *Needed: A Career Ladder in Nursing.* Am. J. Nursing, *68*:6:1234, June, 1968.

Smith, Dorothy M.: *Myth and Method in Nursing Practice.* Am. J. Nursing, *64*:2:68, Feb., 1964.

Speed, Eunice, and Young, Nancy A.: *SCAN—Data Processed Printouts of a Patient's Basic Care Needs.* Am. J. Nursing, *69*:1:108, Jan., 1969.

Statement of Nursing Education by Board of Directors of NLN. Feb., 1967. Nurs. Outlook, *15*:6:12, June, 1967.

The Plight of the U.S. Patient. Time, Feb. 21, 1969, pg. 53.

The Surgeon General Looks at Nursing. Am. J. Nursing, *67*:1:64, Jan., 1967.

The Vanishing Nurse. (Letter) Am. J. Nursing, *67*:1:48, Jan., 1967.

Trites, David K.: *These Myths Hurt Nursing Performance.* Modern Hospitals, *114*:1:90, Jan., 1970.

Unrealistic and Impractical. (Letter) Nurs. Outlook, *15*:2:24, Feb., 1967.

Wiedenbach, Ernestine: *The Helping Art of Nursing.* Am. J. Nursing, *63*:11:54, Nov., 1963.

Young, Lucie S.: *Nursing's Challenge.* Nurs. Outlook, *17*:5:63, May, 1969.

PART TWO

MANAGING YOURSELF
AND OTHERS

I keep six honest serving-men
(They taught me all I knew);
Their names are What and Why and When
and How and Where and Who.

from The Elephant's Child, Stanza I,
by Rudyard Kipling

Chapter 3

Understanding People

Because of our concern for the patient, his needs and his problems, we sometimes forget that our coworkers are human beings, not unfeeling robots, and that all of us have needs that must be satisfied. We can understand the problems and emotions of our patients only to the degree that we understand ourselves and the vital part that the satisfaction of our basic needs plays in the development of each one of us as individuals.

PEOPLE AND THEIR NEEDS

Maslow's hierarchy of needs* suggests that an individual operates on ascending levels in which the needs on one level must be at least partially met before the person is ready to consider the needs on a higher level. The basic level is concerned with the physiological or survival needs, consisting of food, water, oxygen, rest, and so forth. Your coworkers will be able to satisfy these needs themselves, but occasionally problems arise to the extent that they may interfere with their work performance, e.g., hunger due to an omitted breakfast or to a late lunch, or perhaps loss of sleep because of illness in the family or even a late date.

The Need for Recognition. Every person wants to be recognized as an individual, a person with certain abilities as well as with certain limitations. Everyone wants to feel that he or she is important to someone else. Normally, this need for recognition results in certain forms of behavior. For example, creativeness, possessiveness,

---

*Maslow, A. H.: *Motivation and Personality*. Harper and Row Publishers, Inc., New York, 1954.

mastery, rivalry, and display stem from the fact that the human being is motivated to project his ego upon his immediate surroundings.

This desire to be somebody is healthy as long as it remains within normal limits, but if it becomes exaggerated, the individual becomes overly concerned with self and less concerned with others. He becomes selfish, boastful, overcritical, and forgetful of the feelings of others. He seeks in every possible way to draw attention to himself. The words *I, me,* and *mine* play a very important part in his conversation as well as in his thinking.

As a nurse you can use to advantage this need for personal recognition by giving praise and showing appreciation whenever they are deserved. Sincere praise makes the person feel worthwhile and important, stimulating her to continue her good work. Praise is like salt—a little, wisely used, brings out the good qualities; too much spoils them. Sometimes all that is necessary is a simple "thank you," spoken directly to a member of your staff, showing that you recognize her intentions and are grateful for her help.

On the other hand, you will need to control the individual who shows signs of wanting too much attention. The desire for recognition is related to, and dependent upon, other needs. It is possible that one or more of these are not being met to her satisfaction although her behavior seems to point to one area only. Study the individual carefully. Analyze her responses in various situations in an effort to determine their cause. Show appreciation for her satisfactory behavior and, whenever possible, ignore that which is less commendable, thus indirectly helping her to behave in a more acceptable manner.

You must control your own desire to feel important, lest it overshadow the consideration you should give to your staff and thus destroy your effectiveness as a leader.

Nursing students and staff nurses alike complain, "No one pays any attention to us when we do things right, only when we do something wrong." In many cases their complaint is justified because someone forgot their need for recognition and a feeling of self-worth.

The Need To Belong.   Every individual desires to be part of a group. This goes beyond merely wanting to be with people. We are all naturally gregarious, but if the need to belong is to be satisfied, we must feel that we are accepted by others and that they like us. The individual wishes to feel accepted by the entire group because, through this affiliation, he gains the prestige that is accorded to the group as a whole.

This desire to belong is demonstrated most vividly by the teenager and his gang or her crowd. As evidence of belonging, everyone must dress alike, speak alike, have the same mannerisms. We find this group-consciousness just as strong among those adults who join lodges and clubs of all kinds.

In a hospital or nursing home many individuals share in caring for the patient—some directly, some indirectly—but each one is very important to the welfare of each patient. How many of us would be able to, or would care to, go to the engine room and maintain the equipment there so that our patients would have light, heat, and hot water? How many of us would care to wash and iron all the linen for our patients, or to prepare all their food, or do all the cleaning? There was a time when this work was considered a normal part of the nurse's duties. But not any more. Now many persons work together to provide for the comfort and well-being of the patient, and no single worker is more important than another.

In the hospital, uniforms often designate the status of the worker. Thus, we have dietary workers wearing one color, housekeeping workers wearing another, and nursing students still another—each color a badge of belonging to a particular group. Sometimes this organization takes on all the aspects of a caste system in which each individual associates with or feels at ease with only the other members of her own work-group. Usually, in this kind of atmosphere, there is very little mutual understanding or rapport among the various groups.

On the nursing unit every person giving care to the patients is important to each patient. The head nurse must insure that each person's skills and abilities are used in the proper way. Using the word *our* instead of *my* and *your* will help to emphasize that each person is an important member of the group. Your help, encouragement, and example are necessary so that each person realizes that you want her and need her.

Occasionally, you may find a person who does not seem to feel this need to belong. She appears to prefer to work and be alone. She does not readily enter into group conversations. She may even act disdainful of the others, giving the impression that she thinks she is better than they. This behavior may be only a defense. Actually, she may want to be a member of the group, but because she is afraid that they do not want her, she hides behind her seeming wish to be left alone. You will need to encourage and provide opportunities for her to participate in group activities. In addition, you should suggest that other people include her in their conversations, and that they ask for her help, offering to help her in return.

The Need for Understanding. Everyone wants to express herself so that others will understand her and her problems, limitations, fears, hopes, and desires. The need to understand others is just as great. Each person wants to know what others expect of her, what her responsibilities are, and how well she is meeting those responsibilities.

This need for understanding is closely related to the need for recognition since both are based on respect and admiration. We want to be looked up to; yet it is just as important that we ourselves have someone to whom we can look for help and understanding.

Problems are bound to arise if this need is ignored. If one believes that it is unnecessary to understand others, she is likely to become cold, aloof, and uninterested in others and their problems. On the other hand, when there is no desire to be understood, one may become uncommunicative, displaying very little emotion, apparently caring little about the reactions of others toward herself.

If this need to understand and be understood is exaggerated, the person may become so anxious to gain respect that she will seek to obtain it by any means. She may become demanding, expect to have her opinion consulted often, and be excessively anxious to please for fear others will not respect her. She may spend much time discussing the problems of others, give praise lavishly, or become too lenient and overly tolerant of their work and actions in the hope that this will make them like her more.

As a nurse you have an important part in satisfying the needs of other people. Yet your ability to satisfy them is dependent upon your own ability to understand and to be understood. If you feel sorry for yourself, believing that no one understands you and your problems, your loneliness and resentment will be passed on to your staff. They, in turn, will feel that you do not understand them or their problems. You must take an individual interest in each person, seeking to learn the meaning of what they leave unsaid as well as of what they say. Help them to know exactly what they are to do, then let them know how well they are meeting your expectations. If they are not measuring up, determine why; perhaps a need for better understanding exists.

The Need for Stimulation and Personal Growth. Change is stimulating. Change may also be a means of providing a person with the opportunity, as well as the incentive, to acquire new knowledge and understanding, to think new thoughts, to solve more difficult problems, or to learn new skills. Without this stimulation comes boredom, and with boredom comes lack of interest in doing a good job.

The amount of stimulation needed by each individual will vary from person to person, but usually the desire to have some new experiences is always present. Some people will try constantly to see and do new things and will become unhappy when forced to perform "routine" tasks day after day. Other individuals feel more content when their duties entail the performance of the same activities over and over. Such a person may have either a limited intelligence or feelings of inferiority and insecurity. In either case, she is very likely to become upset and unhappy when confronted with new situations.

Providing opportunities to satisfy the desire for personal growth in the various members of your staff is one of the challenging aspects of nursing leadership. You must plan carefully and give close supervision to those individuals who, in their eagerness for new experiences, may thoughtlessly engage in activities that, for the safety of the patient, they should not do. You will need to use all your powers of persuasion to help such persons understand the importance of "routine" tasks in relation to total patient care and will need to show them ways of increasing their experience and skill while performing these duties. Nursing students (and some graduate nurses too) sometimes become bored with giving baths because they feel that other aspects of patient care are so much more exciting and important. They need your help to understand that the importance is not in the giving of the bath itself but in providing a time for the patient to talk out his problems with someone who is capable of helping him.

You must encourage the person who needs new experiences in order to increase her learning and skills. Provide her with the opportunity to•perform a single new activity along with her usual work. Give her the necessary help and moral support for performing this task; make the experience a satisfying one by assuring a successful performance through proper preparation and supervision. Do not forget to praise her when she is finished. Soon you will find that you have a dependable person who can assume much more responsibility.

Occasionally, you may find that you must work with a person who is intellectually incapable of performing more than routine tasks. In this case, you should organize your work in such a way that you make full use of this person's abilities, thereby giving others more time to perform the more complex duties.

The Need for Security. The need for security involves job, group, and spiritual security along with personal security or safety. Everyone must be able to depend upon something or someone, to predict with reasonable accuracy what will happen to her, and to know how others feel toward her. In other words, she must have that comfortable feeling of security if she is to function to her fullest capacity. This feeling of security is the end result of meeting and satisfying the need for recognition, for belonging, for understanding, and for new experiences. The person who feels secure can meet the problems of life with equanimity and can work out acceptable solutions to these problems with a minimum amount of frustration.

PEOPLE AND THEIR FEELINGS AND
ATTITUDES

Feelings may be pleasant or unpleasant and are the result of a person's response either to her environment or to something that happens with herself. Feelings so intense that they affect the internal organs, resulting not only in a mental reaction but in a physical one as well, are called emotions.

When a person's basic needs are satisfied, there is a feeling of pleasure, happiness, and enthusiasm. The person is at peace with herself and with the world. Minor annoyances fail to disturb her since she is able either to shrug them off or to face and overcome them.

If a person's needs are ignored or are not met to her satisfaction, she experiences an unpleasant feeling, which may become so intense that it becomes an emotion, such as anger, jealousy, hate, fear, or discouragement. When this occurs, her response to her immediate surroundings is also affected. Often she will vent her emotions upon someone who had nothing to do with starting this chain reaction. For example, a nurse, when reprimanded by a doctor because a patient did not receive a treatment as directed, was unable to assert herself with the doctor. Instead, she vented her feelings of frustration and anger upon another member of the staff, thereby restoring somewhat her feeling of self-worth.

You must keep in mind that your own emotional responses, along with those with whom you work, will have a profound effect upon the quality of nursing care that they give. You must try to provide situations that will give them a feeling of pleasure. You should also try either to minimize those situations that will result in feelings of frustration or other unpleasant emotions, or to help the person understand and control her reactions to the situation.

Many of your feelings and reactions are the result of, either consciously or unconsciously, learned behavior. These reactions are called attitudes. You do not usually develop them in response to rational or critical thinking based on fact, but rather acquire them through your past experiences in your social environment. You have acquired attitudes toward many things—food, religion, politics, strikes, nationalities, war, team nursing, supervisors, office workers, janitors, farmers, practical nurses, etc. Have your beliefs come about because you collected all available facts, did your own critical thinking, then decided what you wanted to believe about each other?

One instructor had her beginning students fill out a questionnaire after they had had several weeks of classroom and clinical experience. Some of the answers showed that, in spite of classroom instruction related to attitudes toward patients, students seemed to retain many of the attitudes that they had had before entering nursing. One question asked what effect the education, age, place in the family, or wealth of a patient would have on the nursing care that the student would give. Following are some of the answers:

"A person who has no schooling is a moron."

"People who are educated are easier to get along with."

"Old people are inclined to be bossy."

"The youngest in a family is more demanding."

"The father is bossy. He wants more attention and must be made to realize that he is under the staff here and must do as we say."

"I would give a wealthy person more attention because he is used to having more."

Some of these attitudes show definite evidences of biased thinking, yet these students are probably no different from some members of your staff. You should try to identify your own attitudes about various people, about team nursing, and about taking the responsibility for planning and directing patient care. Determine whether or not your attitudes are valid, since they will influence your leadership and your ability to get along with your coworkers.

PEOPLE ARE NOT ALL ALIKE

Although in many respects all human beings are similar, physically, emotionally, and spirtually, no two are exactly alike. There are differences in physical appearances, in emotional responses, and in spiritual beliefs as well as in abilities.

The Ability To Learn.   People differ greatly in their ability to learn. Because of her inherent intelligence, one person may learn a great quantity of material very quickly, while another can learn only a small amount.

The mere fact that a person "learns," i.e., can repeat verbatim a certain amount of information, should not be construed to mean that she has learned it to the point of retaining it for more than a short time. Regardless of the learning process used, a certain amount of material will be forgotten and this amount will differ from person to person. Furthermore, the person who thinks of rote memorization as learning makes another serious mistake. True learning employs logical thinking and association of ideas, i.e., looking for meanings and relationships and combining them into a meaningful unit. Some people find it very easy to memorize words but find it difficult to associate ideas.

The Ability To Apply Knowledge.   Closely related to the ability to see relationships and associate ideas is the ability to apply knowledge. The transference of knowledge into action is perhaps the most difficult skill a nursing student must acquire. It is easy to learn what to do in a particular situation, but change that situation ever so slightly, and the student who has only rote memory to fall back on is lost. Along with knowledge, it is also necessary to attain an understanding of basic principles and methods of applying those principles.

One morning a nursing student was assigned the care of two patients—one recovering from an appendectomy and the other suffering from a coronary thrombosis. The head nurse went over the orders for each patient but gave no further explanation to the student. Sometime later during her rounds, the head nurse found each patient giving his own bath. Calling the student aside, the head nurse asked what principle was important in the treatment of most patients suffering from heart disturbances. The student answered that bed rest was important for them. She knew the doctor's order but did not understand the underlying principles. She saw no relationship between bed rest, rest needed by the heart, and the exertion that the patient experienced while giving his own bath. To this student bed rest meant only keeping the patient in bed.

The Ability To Use One's Hands and Body. This area includes grace, dexterity, and correct body mechanics. Some people learn readily how to make their movements graceful and effective and how to go smoothly from one motion to another. Others handle equipment and their own bodies awkwardly, with much wasted time, motion and energy. Some learn by experience, through trial and error, to achieve at least some degree of dexterity and ease of motion; others seem never to be able to attain it.

The Ability To Control or Display Emotions. To a great extent the outward show of emotion seems to be a learned behavior. The child is told, "Don't cry. You're a big girl now." So, gradually, the child learns to keep many emotions from showing outwardly. Someone says to a nursing student, "Be professional." Somewhere she acquires the idea that being professional in appearance is synonymous with acting impersonally, suppressing one's feelings in order to achieve a cool, calm, impersonal bedside manner. On the other hand, some people frequently show their emotions outwardly; some may even exaggerate them. It is possible to achieve a happy balance between the two extremes.

We need to look beyond the similarities and dissimilarities of people, and to try to understand the distinctions between people. Too often we think that there is one best way for doing something— the way *we* do it; one best way for thinking—the way *we* think; one best way for feeling—the way *we* feel; one way of reacting—the way *we* react. To become an effective leader and get along with people, we have to understand their abilities and their limitations. In other words, we have to see them as unique individuals.

THE IMPORTANCE OF EFFECTIVE COMMUNICATION

In order to get along with people, we must be able to communicate with them and make ourselves clearly understood. Communication is necessary to use the techniques of leadership. The more effective a leader's communication, the more effective will be her leadership.

What is Communication? Communication is more than just saying words. It is the ability to convey ideas and meanings to another person. We have all heard the saying, "Your actions speak so loudly, I can't hear what you say." So it is with our communication. What we do and how we do it convey just as much meaning as what we say; in fact, *what* we say may be less important than *how* we say it. The tone of voice, choice of word, facial expressions and gestures may communicate our ideas and feelings more effectively sometimes than the actual words we use.

To be really effective, communication must be an interchange of ideas. What we say is less important than what people think we are saying; we must make certain that we are putting our ideas across. Not only must we try to make ourselves understood but we must also be open-minded, trying to understand others and their ideas and suggestions.

Communication may be either directive or creative. It is directive when the nurse assigns duties, gives definite information, or demonstrates how to perform a procedure. She uses creative communication when she helps someone determine what should be done and how to do it, or when she listens to someone talk over a personal problem.

How Do We Communicate? Good communication begins with a clear idea about what one wants to say and how to say it. The English language is very complex; a single word may have many meanings, sometimes similar, sometimes dissimilar. A classic example of this is the difference in the meaning that the word *void* conveys to a bookkeeper and to a nurse. *Normal* has a different meaning for a chemist than it does for a biologist, a mathematician, or a psychologist. The word *careful* has at least eight different shades of meaning, while the word *see* has at least twenty. The context of the sentence may indicate the meaning of the word, or the meaning may be inferred from the inflection of the speaker's voice.

As in every profession or trade, hospital workers have their own terminology and jargon, which are, for the most part, extremely puzzling to the uninitiated. Nursing students and new aides quickly pick up this new language and use it as a badge of belonging. Thus cath., prep., O.R., I.V., I.M., trach. care, E.K.G., ad lib, and many others creep into the conversation with patients as well as with other hospital personnel. It seems so easy for the nurse to say to a patient, "Have you been prepped for your g.i. studies tomorrow?" In fact, one nursing student went so far as to chart, "Pt. went to B.R. for B.M. before the lab came to do her B.M.R."

Certain terms and abbreviations are acceptable; however, we should never overuse them nor include them in our conversations with patients. Terminology that seems very commonplace to us can be confusing and frightening to the patient or an inexperienced nursing aide. We must be able to select the word that not only conveys our meaning in the best way, but is also one which is familiar to our listeners. If a word is unfamiliar, then we must define it in terms that the listener can understand.

Not only is communication carried on through the use of words but also by means of the tone or inflection of the voice. For example, take the simple word *yes*. By changing the inflection one may express simple agreement, agreement and sympathy, question, disgust or irritation, ridicule, or astonishment. In addition, gestures and facial expressions convey information about one's feelings. Nodding one's head may indicate agreement, interest, and/or sympathy; raising an eyebrow may show doubt. Words do not need to be used in order to communicate with others.

Another method of conveying ideas is by means of the written word. We communicate through written assignments, reports, and charts. Belonging to a profession implies a certain quality and quantity of education. Yet professional nurses sometimes demonstrate a surprising lack of knowledge about correct grammar and spelling.

As stated previously, facial expressions and gestures convey ideas. In like manner, the use of visual aids to illustrate the ideas we are trying to put across is an effective means of communication. The demonstration of a certain technique or procedure is much more effective than a verbal description only. Put the two together and it becomes easier to put the idea across.

What we do is observed by others. Our actions demonstrate our attitudes and depths of understanding more effectively than all the talking we do. Those who work with us will judge our actions and assume that, since we are professional nurses, the way in which we do our work must be the correct and best way.

You must remember that good communication is necessary for understanding and for cooperation and unified action. Communication, to be effective, must move toward you as well as from you. You must be able to put yourself and your ideas across. On the other hand, you must provide the opportunity for, and seek to understand, communication by others.

How Well Do We Try To Understand Others? Most of us have a tendency to talk too much and listen too little. When trying to find out what others think and believe, we should try to keep our questions and comments brief and to the point. As the old jingle puts it:

> A wise old owl lived in an oak.
> The more he saw, the less he spoke;
> The less he spoke, the more he heard.
> Why can't we be like that wise old bird?

In order to understand others, we must learn to listen with an open mind. To do this we must learn to control our feelings and opinions and become more receptive to those of others. We often think and judge with our feelings; therefore, we must guard against reading our own meaning into what the other person is saying. We cannot afford to jump to a hasty conclusion.

In addition, if we want to understand what we hear, we must be genuinely interested in the other person and in what she is saying. We can display that interest by our expressions, questions, and comments, and by providing the opportunity for others to express themselves.

The ability to understand what another person is saying goes far beyond the recognition of the words used. It involves trying to understand any display of emotions, attitudes, or prejudices. In addition, it means recognizing that what a person does not say may be as important as what he does say. It is only natural for us to try to "save face" and to protect our egos from being undermined. Therefore, we are likely to sound out those around us to determine whether they will be sympathetic and understanding or critical of our actions, opinions, attitudes, or beliefs. Sometimes we are totally unaware that we are using this method of self-protection. For example, a nurses' aide may remark to the head nurse, "Mr. Smith seems to feel that he can't ask the nurses to help him." Could it be that she also has that feeling but is transferring it to a third person to find out what the nurse's reaction might be? Perhaps, if we show more interest in and sympathy for our patients, our coworkers will feel freer to ask for help or to express their opinions and ideas.

Common Barriers to Good Understanding.   Probably the most common cause of misunderstanding is found in our own preconceived ideas, opinions, and beliefs. We are sometimes unable to evaluate facts objectively, because we interpret them with our feelings in the light of our past experience. In doing so we may use false logic. For example, we may believe that:

People who are shifty-eyed do not tell the truth. — Major premise.

Mary Jones is shifty-eyed. — Minor premise.

Therefore, Mary Jones is not telling the truth. — Conclusion.

Our major premise is based upon our belief, which is not a proven fact; therefore, our conclusion may be incorrect. However, our dislike of Mary Jones has begun and, regardless of the circumstances, which may later disprove our original opinion of her, we will have difficulty in overcoming this prejudice. Furthermore, we may communicate our distrust through our actions, and the barrier to mutual understanding grows higher.

Another reason for misunderstanding is found in the fact that we are prone to judge in terms of either right or wrong with no degrees in between. This interpretation is based, as was previously indicated, on our own opinions, ideas, and beliefs, rather than on research and critical analysis of all the available facts. Sometimes we do not even attempt to discover all the facts, or perhaps we are unable or unwilling to consider anyone's viewpoint but our own.

We sometimes behave like the six blind men in the Hindoo fable.* Each went to find out for himself what an elephant looked like. The first man felt the side and decided that the animal was like a wall. The next man happened to feel the tusk, so he was sure that the elephant was like a spear. Still another grabbed the trunk, so he thought the animal was like a snake. The fourth blind man put his arms around the elephant's leg; consequently, to him, the animal was like a tree. The next man felt the elephant's ear, so he compared the animal to a fan. Finally, the last one seized the tail and immediately he thought the elephant was like a rope. Each of the six men clung to his own opinion of what the elephant looked like. Although each man was partly right, each one thought his opinion was the only correct one, and all others were wrong; therefore, no one made any further attempt to find out the truth.

We arrange words into sentences to express ideas. When our grammar is faulty, we have difficulty saying what we mean. The ability of others to understand what we say is, at least in part, dependent upon our ability to place words in their correct relationship to one another. Dangling phrases and indefinite reference or agreement of pronouns will confuse the listener. For example, "having sterilized the instruments, the operation was started" is confusing to say the least. Or suppose you are given this direction, "I'll hold his knee, and when I nod my head, tap it." Would you do as you are told? Using the English language correctly is a necessary part of effective communication.

If we are to be understood, we must speak the language of our listeners. The dangers of misunderstanding arising out of our indiscriminate use of medical terminology and hospital jargon have already been discussed. The mark of an educated person is his ability to speak the language of those around him. Sometimes our desire to

---

*Saxe, John G.: The Blind Men and the Elephant. Home Book of Verse, edited by B. E. Stevenson, Vol. 1, pg. 1877. Henry Holt & Company, Inc., 1940.

demonstrate our knowledge of a subject leads us to use difficult words and lengthy explanations; consequently, what we are saying does not mean much to our listeners. The simpler we make our language, the more likely we are to be understood.

The use of abstract terms and ideas in place of specific words and definitions is still another reason for misunderstandings. Perhaps we are mentally lazy; at any rate, we do not always define clearly in our own minds just what we are trying to say; therefore, others do not understand us well. Abstract terms will be given more concrete meanings by the other person. Thus *small* may mean a drop, a part of a teaspoonful, an entire teaspoonful, a pinch, one piece, a number of pieces, and so on. *Some, large,* a *few* minutes, *don't overdo,* and *just routine* are examples of abstract words and phrases that may mean different things to different people.

Other factors also contribute to our being misunderstood. The listener must be interested if he is to grasp the entire meaning. We can never assume that our listener understands what we are saying. We must always watch for the puzzled expression or frown and try to clarify the point immediately to the satisfaction of all concerned.

How Can You Communicate More Effectively? Think before you speak. Determine what you want to say and how you can say it so that it will be easily understood by others. Be brief and choose your words with care; make each one count.

Mean what you say. Remember that your tone of voice, facial expression, and actions must be in harmony with the content of your message, emphasizing its meaning rather than detracting from it. Put the message in personal terms directed for the personal use of the listener. However, you must talk *with* rather than *at,* and certainly never *down to,* your listener. The pronoun, *I,* should be used less often than *we.* The pronoun, *you,* encourages personal application by directive suggestion, whereas *we* suggests togetherness or belonging. When used properly, each pronoun can contribute to putting across your ideas more effectively.

State your facts objectively. However, you must keep in mind the importance of the other person's emotions in relation to what you are saying. Whenever possible, use a combination of methods of communication—visual as well as verbal—in order to emphasize what you say. Define key terms, then follow with illustrations that are familiar to your listener. Always start with the familiar and proceed to the unknown. Choose definite and specific words rather than abstract ones. In addition, keep in mind the importance of understanding others. Try to evaluate objectively all that you see and hear.

The Art of Gentle Persuasion. We can see the use of persuasion all around us every day. Advertising is one of the most common forms. Teaching also uses persuasion. The books and newspapers we read, the pictures we look at, the conversations we engage in—most, if not all, are directed toward persuading us more or less subtly to believe something and to translate our beliefs into action.

Persuasion is an important activity in leadership, for through persuasion you get a person to do or to believe something because she wants to do or to believe it. Listening is one of the first steps in persuasion. Find out what a person believes and why she believes it. Don't argue or contradict. Ask one or two questions to which the person can answer "Yes." Make one or two suggestions. Avoid those words suggesting ideas against which she has already indicated prejudice. Make your ideas attractive. Show the person how much she will benefit from following your ideas. (This is a basic principle in advertising. "Feel good again with . . . tonic!" or "Want to look your best? Wear a . . . girdle.") Later, the person may offer your original idea as if it was hers from the very beginning. This is the result of effective persuasion. Now she will believe in that idea because it is hers.

Rumors and What To Do about Them.   Almost always rumors are caused by a lack of communication. Much has been said about the hospital grapevine. When people feel that they have not been told everything, they will quickly supply their own reasons. Sometimes they would rather believe a false statement than a true one, because it is what they want to believe. Rumors are also caused by a misunderstanding somewhere along the line of communication or by the prejudices and personal opinions of a listener.

Preventing rumors is better than trying to stop them after they have been started; therefore, you must keep your staff well-informed concerning changes in hospital policies and the reasons for these changes. No rumor should be ignored, for it indicates that the line of communication has become blocked somewhere. Get all the available facts and pass them on to your coworkers as soon as possible.

GIVING PEOPLE A "PSYCHOLOGICAL PAYCHECK"

The phrase, "psychological paycheck," is borrowed from industry. Occasionally we hear people say, "I wouldn't work there if they paid me ten times what I'm getting now," or "I wouldn't do that for a million dollars." What they are saying is that a job must give something more than a mere monetary return for their time. People must like their work and the people they work with. In other words, they want to receive a psychological paycheck—job satisfaction.

Job satisfaction comes with being able to do good work and knowing that it is recognized and appreciated. Satisfaction comes if credit is given freely when credit is due and criticism is given fairly when needed. People want to know what they are supposed to do and how they are measuring up to the expectations of their co-workers and their superiors.

Job satisfaction comes with mutual respect between people — respect for each person as an individual and for his capabilities. Emerson once said, "Every man I meet is in some way my superior. In that, I learn of him."

Effective management starts with understanding people and helping them understand you. Only when you try to understand yourself and the methods you use to satisfy your own needs will you be able to give to others that intangible reward called a psychological paycheck.

STUDY QUESTIONS

1. Determine a satisfactory criterion to guide you in giving recognition and praise.
2. Do you think that the wearing of different colored uniforms by the various hospital work-groups is good? Give your reasons.
3. How could you direct your staff without giving them the impression that you feel that they are working *under* you?
4. Look for situations in which a person's feelings and emotions may have affected her work.
5. What is your attitude toward each of the following? Analyze how your attitude developed. Is your attitude valid and why?
   a. A head nurse, a supervisor, a practical nurse, a nurses' aide, and a nursing student.
   b. A rich patient, a patient from a slum district, a hippie.
   c. A patient who is a Jew, a Negro, a Mexican, a Russian, or an American Indian.
   d. A patient who is a college president, a doctor, an office worker, a ditch digger, a policeman, a garbage collector.
   e. A patient who is elderly, an infant, a child, a teen-ager, a young adult, a patient in his fifties.
   f. A person who is an alcoholic, who smokes marijuana or takes LSD or "pep pills," or who smokes three to four packs of cigarettes daily.
6. What do you mean when you use the following expressions: in a minute, don't worry, just a routine specimen, "clean" and "dirty" cases, float nurse, scrub nurse, neurotic? How might each one be interpreted by a patient, by a new nursing student, by an inexperienced nursing assistant?
7. Observe on the hospital unit for illustrations of communication (verbal and nonverbal) that were or could have been misunderstood by one of the persons involved. What should be done to improve the understanding?
8. Make a list of abstract words or phrases that a nurse commonly uses. How can each be made more specific in meaning?
9. Trace one rumor. Determine, if possible, its cause and how it could have been prevented.
10. Discuss what you want in a job in order to receive job satisfaction.
11. How can you encourage or persuade a person to change his ideas or beliefs? Select a person and try to change his beliefs about something. How successful were you? Why?

Chapter 4

Leadership in Administration

The term leadership is in itself difficult to define, since it contains broad concepts, which vary according to the person who is using the word. Sometimes it is easier to define the term by indicating the traits of a leader or the results of leadership.

SOME DEFINITIONS

Funk and Wagnalls' *Standard Dictionary* defines *leadership* as the "position of a leader; guidance," and the verb *to lead* as "to go with or ahead of so as to show the way; guide."

Certainly leadership implies the presence of other people and a relationship between those people and the person who is leading. Where there is a leader there must be followers. However, mere appointment to the position of leader does not in any way insure that he will be accepted by the group, nor does it imply that he is capable of giving leadership. A leader must possess those qualities which enable him to make people want to accomplish something. "Leadership does not mean domination. . . . The leader's job is to get work done by other people, . . . in getting people to work for you when they are under no obligation to do so. . . . No matter what point we start from in a discussion of leadership we inevitably reach the conclusion that the art of being a leader is the art of developing people."*

---

*Used with permission from *About Being a Leader* in the Monthly Letter published by the Royal Bank of Canada, October 3, 1957.

GENERAL TYPES OF LEADERSHIP

Directive Leadership. One kind of leadership is *directive,* sometimes called *autocratic.* Directive leadership in its most extreme form implies a dictator who is arbitrary and prejudiced, insisting that his is the only right way and allowing no argument, logical or otherwise, to sway him from the goal and the methods that he has selected.

In a more modified form, directive leadership combines fairness with firmness, kindliness with decisiveness, respect for the individual with power over the individual. The person using directive leadership considers himself in a position of authority, and expects his followers to respect him and to obey his directions. He may listen to suggestions, but he is not necessarily influenced by them. He has set his goals and expects them to be accepted along with his methods of achieving them. He knows what has to be accomplished and believes that he knows the best way to get it done. He does not encourage individual initiative or even cooperation between the various members of the group.

While directive leadership is not always the best form of leadership, it is necessary in cases of emergency or crisis, when there is no time for a group to decide on a plan of action. It is also useful when the leader is the only one who has new and essential information or skills, or when the members of the group are inexperienced. Also the leader must use a more directive approach when the workers expect to be told what to do, or when a worker is unsure of himself or his ability to do something on his own.

Creative Leadership. Another kind of leadership is *creative.* Here a democratic atmosphere emphasizes "togetherness." Under this form of leadership the workers are informed of the overall purposes and progress of the entire organization and of their own relationship within this organization. Each one is made to feel that he has an important contribution to make. The leader guides the workers in selecting acceptable goals and in determining an effective plan of action to achieve those goals. He allows them to make certain decisions for themselves, although he guides and helps them; consequently, they have a greater feeling of satisfaction and freedom. Creative leadership is implied in the definition, "to go with or ahead of so as to show the way."

Lao-tse, a Chinese philosopher, who lived a few hundred years before the birth of Christ, suggests that a good leader exerts his leadership in such a way that his followers do not realize that he exists, rather they believe that they did the work by themselves. The democratic leader works through people, not by domination, but by suggestion and persuasion. The more successful he is in the use of human relations, the greater is his influence as a leader. The honor and satisfaction which he receives will not come from the public acclaim, but rather from the knowledge that his goals are reached and the work is well done.

An extreme form of democratic leadership exists when the leader allows too much worker domination of activities with too little guidance, or when he permits the workers to do as they please until at last there is no guidance at all. This is sometimes described as "laissez faire" leadership. This let-alone policy will repudiate any leadership that may have been present at the beginning, and the work situation will rapidly disintegrate into a disorganized hodge-podge in which no one knows what he is supposed to do, nor does he care. A worker in this kind of atmosphere will lose all sense of initiative and desire for achievement. There is no place in nursing for this kind of nonleadership.

Results of Leadership. The leader's primary purpose is to keep the group headed in the right direction. He must also decide what approach will be most effective in keeping the group constantly moving forward. But whatever the approach, effective leadership must bring results that are consistent with the aims of the organization.

While it is not easy to define leadership, it is easy to measure it in terms of what has been accomplished. Effective leadership brings several results: a spirit of cooperation and enthusiasm based on good human relationships; well-trained, skilled workers, and an efficiently run organization, able to meet its goals. In other words, good leadership improves job performance.

LEADERSHIP IN ADMINISTRATION

Leadership is needed in every area of nursing. The departmental administrator, the supervisor, the head nurse, and the staff nurse must all be leaders, each in her particular field. The professional nurse in the hospital today is finding that she is moving away from the bedside of the patient because she must assume more and more administrative duties. This does not mean that she can become any the less concerned about patient care. It does mean that, in addition to being able to give good nursing care, she must be able to direct others in giving that care. Working with and through people is a necessary part of her leadership.

What Is Administration? Administration is the directing of a group, large or small, in its various activities so that it can reach its over-all aims in the most effective way. It sets up its goals, policies, and procedures so that all personnel can work toward the same goals. In any large group these over-all aims are made more specific in the aims of each subdivision or department, although the point of emphasis will vary according to the specific responsibilities delegated to the department. Good management in any area demands that definite lines of responsibility be set up through which the delegation of duties may be made along with the necessary authority to ensure their proper completion. Management involves all activities necessary to achieve the aims of the organization (in nursing, good patient care) through the efficient use of time, energy, equipment, materials, and the capabilities of every worker. Effective management results in the cooperation of all personnel in working toward a common goal.

Every administrator and manager must exercise leadership. Conversely, any leader will engage in administrative activities. An administrator guides and directs a group or an organization toward a selected goal, and a nurse becomes an administrator by virtue of the guidance and direction which she gives her coworkers; therefore, both the administrator and the head nurse and even the staff nurse must utilize the same principles in order to work with and through people.

Administrative Activities. Effective management is based upon certain principles and must be practiced by everyone who is concerned with directing people—hospital administrator, departmental administrator, supervisor, head nurse, or staff nurse working with auxiliary personnel. The scope and area of practice will be different for each of these persons, but the principles will remain the same.

Definite plans must be formulated that are based upon the objectives, policies, standards, and work procedures previously accepted by the organization. The primary objective of the hospital is caring for the patient. Every department within the hospital enlarges upon some aspect of this over-all aim. The nursing service department is concerned with giving continuous care to the patient. The head nurse and her staff apply those policies, standards, and methods relating to patient care and the evaluation of that care; the nurse and her coworkers plan ways of giving individualized patient care. By planning this care and directing the workers, the nurse is engaging in administrative leadership.

The plans of the organization as a whole must indicate the relationship between each department and the ways in which each must contribute to the achievement of the aims of the organization. In each case these plans must be unified and coordinated by a single individual. The nurse coordinates the activities of her staff. She, in turn, may be responsible to another person who plans and coordinates the work for a larger area.

All personnel and their activities must be systematically arranged so that responsibility and the authority for specific, well-defined duties can be delegated. The hospital organizational charts should show the direct and indirect lines of relationship, while the written policies in job descriptions should define clearly all duties and responsibilities. Lines of communication and the delegation of authority must follow these organizational lines over which a two-way exchange of ideas and information is of vital importance if the entire organization is to function smoothly. This two-way communication includes the administrator's responsibility for delegating functions and the worker's responsibility for reporting about her activities. Although the administrator can and should delegate duties and necessary authority to insure completion of those duties, she cannot delegate her responsibility and must insure that all work meets acceptable standards both in quality and in quantity.

On the nursing unit the professional nurse plans the nursing care of her patients and directs her staff by making assignments and delegating certain parts of the patient's care. A ward manager would perform those administrative activities related to running the unit smoothly and efficiently, thus allowing the head nurse time to be directly concerned with her staff and the care of her patients. There is a trend toward giving her a different title in order to eliminate the old-fashioned idea that a head nurse sits at the desk. She may be called head nurse of nursing care, nursing care coordinator, or even team leader.

An adequate number of qualified personnel is necessary to carry out the plans and achieve the aims of the organization. The qualifications of each person will vary according to the demands of the jobs she is to do, yet each one must realize that she has a definite and important place within the framework of the organization.

To borrow a phrase from industry, "too many chiefs and not enough Indians" indicates poor administrative policies; on the other hand, a sufficient number of qualified chiefs must be available to insure good leadership for the Indians. It is impractical to insist that one group is more important than the other, for each is dependent upon the other if the goals of the organization are to be achieved. A hospital unit, if it is to give adequate care to its patients, must have sufficient administrative persons as well as professional nurses and other personnel who are more directly concerned with caring for the patients. However, people with administrative responsibilities must be qualified to provide the leadership necessary for getting the work completed in an organized, effective way. All persons must be qualified to perform those duties assigned to them.

Administration must use each person's capabilities effectively. This principle involves the use of tools of management, such as human relations and personnel management and supervision, in order to meet the needs of the individual and to give each person adequate satisfaction in her job. Good administration considers the abilities and differences of the individual, then tries to place her in the job that best suits her capabilities. No matter how many workers are available, the work will not get done, the patients will not receive care, unless the administrator or leader is able to use each person effectively. Very little patient care will be given under the "laissez faire" form of leadership.

Frequently, all of the capabilities of an individual are not used because of inadequate planning. The manager must know what each person can do and decide ahead of time where to place each one in order that he can do his best work. Using a worker's capabilities to the fullest extent does not mean that the administrator is a slave driver or that there is exploitation of the worker. It simply means putting the right person in the right job at the right time. Nurses frequently comment about a "well-run station" or a "poorly-run station." Undoubtedly they are referring to the results of well-planned leadership in the one instance and the apparent lack of planning and leadership in the other.

Many of our difficulties in shortage of time result from our inability to use the capabilities of people most effectively according to their job descriptions, or to redefine their job activities to conform with the modern concepts of nursing responsibilities. Very often registered nurses insist that they are the only persons capable of charting, recopying doctors' orders, and doing the other "paper work," yet they think that the nurses' aide is quite capable of caring for a critically ill patient or deciding when a patient should have something for pain.

Cooperative effort is essential to coordinate the activities of the various departments and personnel. Every department and every worker contributes to the care of the patient. No one person should be allowed to consider herself more necessary or important than anyone else. Only when everyone works together harmoniously, making full use of all facilities, can the organization as a whole expect to reach its objectives. This fact is just as true for a group engaged in patient care on a single unit as it is for the hospital as a whole. The patient will benefit only to the extent that everyone gives of her abilities to help the patient. Leadership and teamwork are essential to the smooth functioning of a nursing unit.

However, someone must be responsible for planning ways and means of coordinating the care of the patient. For example, the patient will derive very little benefit if the doctor wants to start an intravenous feeding at the same time the nurses' aide wants to give the bath, the team leader wishes to irrigate a wound, and an x-ray technician wants to take an x-ray. Yet such a situation can develop if the professional nurse fails to plan ahead. There must be a clear understanding, however, concerning who has the final authority to do this planning.

Maximum results must be obtained with a minimum amount of time, effort, supplies, and equipment. The expenditure of money is always of great concern to administration. Economy must be practiced for the benefit of both the hospital and the patient. Unnecessary use of electricity, stationery supplies and linen, coupled with the waste of dressings, drugs, food, etc., all contribute to increased cost of hospitalization to the patient. Budgeting of supplies and care in the use of equipment must be the concern of every hospital employee.

The time and energy used by each worker must result in patient care, otherwise they are being wasted. The nurse must watch for unnecessary motions and steps and try to help her staff use their time and energy as efficiently as possible. She may need to study the causes for needless running back and forth for supplies and equipment, then plan ways for having these essentials available when and where they are needed. She may need to help someone learn how to perform a certain part of a patient's care so that every motion counts.

Wasted time and effort may be dangerous, or at least annoying, to the patient. From the worker's point of view, undue effort may be so tiring that she is unable to care properly for her patients. On the other hand, undue effort by the patient as a result of nursing care awkwardly given may cause serious consequences. Every professional nurse must analyze closely the time and motions involved in giving patient care and must look for more efficient methods. As a whole, nurses are likely to follow procedures or devise short cuts without questioning whether or not those procedures can be improved or if the short cut is safe. Every nurse should be able to plan her work efficiently. Problem-solving and work planning methods will be discussed in more detail in Chapter 5.

Adequate reports must be made and adequate records must be kept. Records and reports contain tangible proof of the effectiveness of the activities of the group and are fundamental to good management. Well-informed people work together more efficiently, are more cooperative, and show greater interest and satisfaction in their own work and in the progress of the organization. A good report is essential for good patient care by the individual worker, and makes administration aware of the problems as well as the progress of all the workers.

Records are written reports, indicating the work completed and nursing problems solved by the group. The patient's chart includes a report of nursing techniques performed and observations made by the staff. The head nurse is concerned with many kinds of records — the patient-condition report, census records, narcotic records, accident reports, time sheets, and others. Some records are legal documents that must be kept on file; other records are valuable for a short time only. Every department within the hospital keeps records concerning its activities. Such records are necessary if administration is to evaluate the progress of the organization.

This brief résumé of the functions of administration should make one aware that managerial and leadership skills and activities are similar. Any person who directs and supervises people must use these administrative functions. The effectiveness of their use is limited only by the capabilities of the individual and the scope of his responsibility.

LEADERSHIP IN SUPERVISION

Since administration delegates duties and responsibilities to the various departments or persons within the organization, supervision becomes a tool of administration to insure the successful completion of these duties. The supervisor must know the aims of administration and must be able to utilize effectively all administrative and leadership functions. In this way, the supervisor complements administration.

What Is Supervision? The word *supervision* conveys different ideas to different people. It is most often believed to be the inspection and checking of a worker's performance in his job by someone who looks only for those things that are being done wrong. In this conception, the emphasis of supervision is placed on getting the work done according to definite policies and procedures. The supervisor plans all the work, makes all the decisions, and issues commands to the workers who are to obey them without question. This is the traditional autocratic form of supervision, which has been practiced in industry and nursing for many years. It stifles both the initiative and the productivity of the individual and seems to think of him as a machine rather than as a human being.

Gradually, however, business and education are changing their ideas about supervision from the dictatorial to a more democratic form. The emphasis, instead of being on getting the work done, is now being placed on helping the individual do his work better. There is a greater degree of democracy and freedom, with the worker being given a voice in the setting up of work goals and planning methods for reaching them. The nursing profession is also beginning to accept these changing concepts of supervision. The implication of team nursing points to the belief that a group of people thinking, planning, and working together with competent supervision can give better nursing care than was possible under the older method of direction.

As with leadership, it is difficult to find a satisfactory definition of supervision, although it is very easy to describe the traits of a good supervisor or to determine the results of supervision. Effective supervision employs techniques from many fields of endeavor — communications, human relations, personnel management, education and others — in order to accomplish its aims. Basically, it deals with people and their personal growth; therefore, as in administration, leadership is fundamental to good supervision.

The quantity and quality of supervision will be determined by the philosophy of the individual and his ability to use the techniques on which supervision is founded. If this individual is overly directive by nature, he is likely to "drive" rather than "lead," resulting in a "do as I tell you" kind of supervision. If the person believes in creative leadership, he will make his supervision more democratic. In one, the supervision given will be direction and inspection; in the other, it will become teaching and helping the worker to develop new skills and a greater understanding of his job.

More democratic supervision is needed in nursing today, but it can be obtained only when nursing leaders believe in the worth and dignity of each person as an individual, and when they become willing to assume the responsibilities inherent in leadership, in administration and supervision. Experience as a leader in team nursing allows the registered nurse to gain experience in the necessary techniques and provides an unlimited field in which to practice the skills demanded by creative leadership.

Purposes of Good Supervision.   Since supervision is concerned with the worker, it must also be concerned with the area where the person works — his working conditions — as well as with the work itself. The supervisor must try to provide, insofar as he is able, suitable working conditions. This involves not only the physical surroundings but also the atmosphere in which the person works. It includes the quantity of supplies and available equipment and the ease with which they can be obtained. The environment in which the person works should give him a feeling of freedom and the desire to do the best he can. The supervisor cultivates a spirt of cooperation, as evidenced by the emphasis on "we" rather than "I." Policies and procedures are formulated by the group, guided by the supervisor.

The supervisor is also concerned with the planning, the execution, and the evaluation of the work to be done. However, the worker, again guided by the supervisor, has a part in this planning and is helped to perform and evaluate his own work. On occasion, the supervisor may need to employ problem-solving techniques and

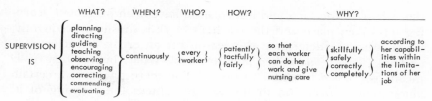

Figure 1.

experiments in order to find better methods for performing the duties delegated to his group; however, he will also seek suggestions from the members of the group.

Although the supervisor is interested in the working conditions and the work being done, his primary concern is for the worker himself. One of the main aims of supervision, if not the principal one, is the orientation, training, and guidance of the individual, based upon his needs and directed toward the utilization of his capabilities and his development of new skills. The supervisor must be acquainted with each individual and be able to stimulate within each person the desire for self-improvement. Then after the person recognizes his need to improve, the supervisor must supply the necessary help and instruction, at the same time guiding the worker in the acquisition of acceptable attitudes, interests, and good work habits.

There is a direct relationship between the help the worker receives and the quality of the care she is able to give. In other words, the care given by nonprofessional workers will be only as good as the help or supervision they receive.

Just as the nonprofessional person needs help to do her job, so also do the staff nurse, the nursing student, the head nurse, and others. In fact, in any position there comes a time when the person needs advice and guidance from someone more experienced than she. Supervision then can be described as *guided learning*.

Supervision Uses Teaching. Supervision in itself is not teaching, yet it must make use of some of the teaching skills as a means of helping the worker. This can be done easily and effectively while the nurse works with her staff.

WHAT IS LEARNING? Learning does not always insure the acquisition of understanding and wisdom. Funk and Wagnalls define *learning* as "the process of getting knowledge," and *knowledge* as "the aggregation of facts and principles, acquired and retained," thus implying that a certain amount of active participation on the part of the learner is necessary. *Wisdom* and *understanding*, on the other hand, imply the ability to put knowledge into practice through the use of judgment and the power to make decisions.

SOME FALLACIES CONCERNING TEACHING. Two fallacies concerning teaching need to be considered. The first involves the belief that when all the facts and information have been presented, learning has taken place and the teacher's work is finished. Frequently, when trying to determine the reason for an error, a teacher may exclaim, "But I *taught* her how to do it!" What this teacher really means is, "I *told* her how to do it." The mere giving of a certain amount of information in no way guarantees the learning of it; learning will not occur unless the learner wishes to acquire that knowledge. Certainly the ability to repeat the information thus acquired does not, in itself, indicate understanding, which is the ability to apply knowledge in a practical way.

Schools of nursing often emphasize the acquisition of knowledge but pay little attention to the degree of understanding that the nursing student acquires or needs. Most examinations in nursing are objective in form and stress recognition of facts, rather than the application of those facts to a particular patient. The so-called situation questions are difficult to make, especially those that will give a valid evaluation of a student's understanding of an actual nursing problem. Yet the acquisition of this understanding is extremely important if we are to have well-prepared nurses, capable of assuming leadership roles in the various nursing fields of endeavor.

A teacher can never assume that what she thinks she has taught and what the student has actually learned are the same. One day while supervising her students, a nursing instructor saw one student bathing a patient who was inadequately draped. The instructor discussed the reasons for draping, and the student indicated her knowledge of the various acceptable methods that could be used. Several days later the teacher came into a room while this same student was again bathing a patient who was incorrectly covered. The student's explanation was, "I didn't think you were coming around today!" The instructor thought she had taught the student to cover all her patients correctly. Actually, the student had learned only that she must cover the patient whenever the instructor was observing her.

Another common fallacy concerns the belief that teaching can be done only in a classroom. Nothing is farther from the truth. Teaching and learning can occur at any time and in any place. Probably one of the most important methods of teaching is by example; people learn from watching and listening to others. Attitudes, ideas, beliefs, even ways of doing things, are passed on from one person to another in this way. The adage, "What you do speaks so loudly I can't hear what you say," is especially true in nursing. Those methods of nursing care that a person observes and practices on the hospital wards will be remembered much longer than the methods described, or even demonstrated, in the classroom. A graduate nurse often says, "I could never be a teacher," yet the staff nurse is one of the most important teachers in nursing today because others will do as they see her do. Many a woman has learned to make a bed correctly while she was a patient in the hospital. Moreover, in nursing, the nursing assistants, L.P.N.'s, and nursing students will watch the registered nurse practitioner, and will follow her example as they care for their patients.

THE RESULTS OF LEARNING. The end result of learning is a change in behavior and may involve mental, emotional, or physical activity. In other words, learning may change either a person's thoughts and ideas, his attitudes, or his ways of doing things. The manifestations of these changes will vary according to the individual's capacity or opportunity for self-expression and will not be noted until a situation arises in which that learning must be used. A person may respond in a certain way because of the teaching he received weeks, months, or even years previously. Learning took place at that time, but the evidence of his learning did not appear until he had occasion to apply his knowledge.

FOUR STEPS TO USE IN TEACHING. As a professional nurse, you will need to apply your entire knowledge of medical therapy and nursing principles as you try to improve the care of your patients. You will need to increase your understanding of people and their reactions, not only of your patients but of your coworkers and of yourself as well. In addition, you will need to use various methods of teaching to help your group to acquire more knowledge and understanding of what good nursing care entails.

The four main steps to effective teaching are *prepare, present, practice,* and *follow-up.* Each step is important and leads naturally into the following one.

Prepare. This includes the preparation of the learner as well as the preparation of yourself as teacher. First of all, you should decide what you want the person to learn. Go over the sequence of points in your own mind or jot them down in the form of a written outline. Make certain that all material is arranged in logical order. You must give some thought also to the prerequisite knowledge that is necessary if the person is to understand what you hope to teach. Decide how you want to present your information. Don't use the same method all the time. Have all the necessary equipment available before you begin. Of course, it goes without saying that you must know your subject.

After you have decided *what* and *how,* you must find out how much the learner knows about the subject already, or what background knowledge she has. For example, it would be difficult to teach someone how to measure output if she does not understand the meaning of cc. or oz. on measuring devices. Start with that which she knows, and proceed to the unknown. Always try to relate the information to what she already understands. Do not assume that because a procedure is routine or the information is simple to you, it will be routine or simple to someone else.

Try to put the person at ease, physically as well as emotionally. External distractions should be minimized as much as possible. At the same time, you should try to show the learner why she needs to know the material being presented and how it will help her in her work. In other words, try to arouse her interest in the subject. Learning occurs with greater rapidity when the learner is receptive, i.e., at ease and interested.

Present. This second step is made up of two parts—telling and showing. Sometimes the discussion may precede the demonstration. Often, however, they are combined into a single operation, but both steps should be used to make your teaching more understandable.

Consider first how to present by telling. Here you must use all the techniques previously discussed in relation to communication— both verbal and nonverbal. Use simple terms that can be understood by the learner. There is no need to show off your complete knowledge of the subject. A good teacher knows how to sort out and use only that information needed by the learner. Giving too much explanation might cause confusion, thereby retarding the learning process.

Make your instruction personal to the learner, repeatedly telling her how she can make use of it. Use illustrations familiar to her, yet ones that are related to the new material being presented. For instance, if you are describing a new method for preventing bedsores, show her how one of her own patients could be helped by this method.

Another important part in the presentation is determining that the person understands what you are telling her, and that she is interpreting what you say correctly. If she does not seem to understand, be patient. Whenever it is necessary to repeat, try a different approach, using different words either to define the terms that were not understood or to restate the information. Technical abbreviations or medical terminology, such as hemiplegia or mediastinum, may not be completely understood by a young nursing student or a nonprofessional person, even though they may use them quite glibly. Unless you are trying to teach the meaning and correct usage of terms, try to avoid using very technical language.

Always put in positive terms those things that the person is expected to do; use the negative, i.e., things not to do, when you want to emphasize precautions necessary for the safety of the patient. In both cases, you should give a brief and simple explanation of the purpose of the procedures or the reasons for the treatment the patient is receiving. It is very important that the person, especially the nonprofessional person, should gain an adequate understanding of the total care that the patient needs.

A seriously injured accident victim, who had a tracheostomy to facilitate suctioning, was admitted to a surgical ward. A nurse asked a nurses' aide to help her in the care of this patient and then instructed her in giving her part of the care. Later the nurse was shocked to overhear this nurses' aide exclaim to another aide, "If I am ever hurt, I don't want to come to this hospital. The first thing they do is slit your throat!" Clearly this aide did not understand the importance of the tracheostomy in the treatment of this patient. Furthermore, she would probably discuss her feelings not only with hospital personnel but also with people outside the hospital, thereby creating a problem in public relations. Perhaps a few additional words by the nurse as the two worked together would have increased the aide's understanding and, consequently, her appreciation of the treatment necessary for this patient.

However, explanation alone is sometimes not enough. Verbal illustrations, while helpful, cannot take the place of visual aids; therefore, demonstration is also an important aspect of teaching, especially in team nursing. The power of your setting the example has already been mentioned and may be described as an informal demonstration of nursing care or behavior that others will observe and perhaps learn. Visual aids definitely help to develop a better understanding of information and foster retention of facts. They may be used to demonstrate ways of giving certain aspects of patient care, or to explain reasons for doing the care in a certain way. Examples of visual aids that you could use to make your teaching more interesting and understandable include pictures, models, sample equipment, or demonstrations of a procedure itself.

When giving a demonstration, go through it slowly, taking one step at a time. Additional explanation should be given throughout, even though you may have given some preliminary information already. Show the easiest way to do the procedure, stressing the precautions and reasons for doing each step. This explanation should not be lengthy nor be given in technical terms. Keep in mind that the simpler the explanation, the easier it will be for the learner to understand and remember it.

Place the learner so that she can see clearly each step of the demonstration and preferably from the same angle as when she does it herself. In other words, if you are teaching someone how to tie a square knot, the person should be watching from behind you rather than facing you, so that your movements and the appearance of the knot will not be reversed.

Allow time for comments and questions. When the procedure is difficult or long, repetition will probably be necessary. The fact that the learner does not ask questions does not always indicate understanding. Sometimes her lack of comprehension is so great that she is unable to ask questions, or she may think she understands when in reality she does not. Therefore, you should ask a few questions yourself to determine if you are getting your information across.

Practice. Doing a procedure, or putting the information into practice, is a necessary step in the learning process. It also gives you the opportunity to check the correctness of the person's learning. At first, this practice must be done under your supervision, the closeness of which will be determined by the past experience of the individual and by the complexity of the procedure. Do not offer too much assistance in the actual performance. It is usually best to suggest the correct method rather than taking over and doing it yourself. For example, you may suggest:

Don't you think it would be easier if . . . ?

Remember there is something else that should be done first.

Do you remember what I did next?

Now stop and think a minute before you do that.

The average person needs several such practice periods in order to develop manual dexterity and to remember the proper sequence of steps necessary for a given procedure. Encourage the learner as she shows improvement and gains in self-confidence. The amount of help and direction may be decreased as the worker shows evidence of learning; however, a certain amount of supervision will always be necessary. You can never leave the learners to practice entirely on their own.

Follow-up. Additional checking at intervals is a necessary and important aspect of teaching. Observe the individual as she performs the entire procedure; look at the finished product; ask some questions to determine if she remembers the reasons for giving the care and the precautions necessary for the safety of the patient. Suggest ways in which she can improve but be very sure to compliment her on the part of her performance that she did well.

This discussion may make the teaching of good nursing care seem lengthy and a somewhat complicated process; however, this is not true. For example, suppose that, as you are passing out medications, you observe a nurses' aide trying to release the side rails on a patient's bed. They are new and somewhat different from the ones previously used, and she is unable to remove them. She is already in a situation that has prepared her for being taught; you need only to introduce your instruction by saying, "Let me help you." Your presentation of the method and its demonstration may consist of, "To lower this side rail, just remove these two pins. This unlocks the rail. Now you can fold it together like this. Then fasten it here so that the rail is out of the way. Just to be safe, always press down on the rail to make sure that it is locked securely." She watches while you lower the rail and lock it in place, then she goes around to the other side of the bed and releases the other rail. This is her practice period. You have taught; she has learned. The time involved was probably not over three minutes.

Perhaps you overhear one of your group saying, "I don't see why we have to get old Mr. Jones up in a chair every day. All we do is lift him from one place to another." Here is a good opportunity to do some teaching by answering the implied question, and thus increasing the understanding of the purpose for this aspect of the patient's treatment in relation to his needs. You can give the information immediately, or you can bring the incident up during the discussion at a nursing care conference so that the entire group will benefit from the explanation.

Teaching, including the subsequent follow-up or observation, is fundamental to good supervision. Each member of your staff must know what she is to do and how to do it. It is your responsibility to give her the opportunity to acquire this knowledge whenever she needs it. Teaching may also be necessary to help the person acquire acceptable attitudes, better appreciation of her contribution to patient care, and a clearer understanding of her responsibility to the patient.

STUDY QUESTIONS

1. Why may some people be autocratic in their direction of other people, while others are democratic?

2. Must a leader be able to perform every task better than any of the workers? State your reasons.

3. Obtain or make an organizational chart for your hospital. Trace the lines of direct and indirect relationships from the main governing body down through the various departments.

4. Determine how the main aims of your hospital are enlarged or made more specific in the objectives of each department.

5. Discuss the statment that supervision may be defined as "guided learning."

6. Discuss the statement, "Practice makes perfect."

7. What specific duties and responsibilities given to the professional nurse can she delegate to someone else? What can she not delegate?

Chapter 5

Leadership in Management

Management is sometimes defined as the effective use of selected methods to accomplish predetermined objectives. It is action with a purpose. In one of their monthly letters a writter for the Royal Bank of Canada says, "If there is any managerial imperative it is summed up in three words: awareness, action, responsibility. These are seen in his handling of problems and dangers and his seeking of goals."* Administration and management are sometimes used interchangeably, but perhaps we would be more correct if we think of management as one process by which administration accomplishes its aims.

One of the definitions of leadership is getting things done through people. A leader can accomplish nothing alone. This is also true of a manager. One of the roles of a nursing leader is that of manager, for she must work *with* and *through* people. She is also concerned with the completion of those activities necessary to the efficient running of a patient unit and achieving the aim of good care for each patient.

MAJOR FUNCTIONS OF MANAGEMENT

The major functions of a manager are planning, organizing, directing, and controlling. *Planning* determines what should be accomplished and how these goals should be reached. *Organizing* arranges the various people, supplies and systems needed to carry out the plans. It includes providing guidelines in the form of policies

---

*"On Being a Manager." The Royal Bank of Canada Monthly Letter. *51*:2:1 (Feb., 1970).

and procedures to help in the work of people in achieving the aims of administration. *Directing* regulates the activities needed to actively carry out the plans with the organized resources made available. *Controlling* evaluates and regulates all of the other functions.

Management Must Solve Problems.   Managerial action is concerned with solving problems; therefore, the nurse who has managerial responsibilities must be willing to accept the challenge of recognizing and thinking through problems in a systematic way. Problems must be solved before the functions of management can be carried out. Frequently planning involves the solving of problems; or better, foreseeing possible difficulties and preventing their occurrence.

Even when you have planned your work carefully, situations may develop that you must straighten out. Your staff know that problems and emergencies do occur. They want a leader who will help them efficiently. Efficiency does not come all at once. It increases with growth in knowledge, understanding, and wisdom. It is never completed; rather, it is a continuous process.

In another letter from the Royal Bank of Canada the writer says, "The adage 'let well enough alone' has no place in the life of a man seeking efficiency. There is no point at which the efficient man can stop and say 'I am.' He goes on to declare 'I am becoming.' . . .

"Of course, we cannot expect to solve every problem, however efficient we may become. We must occasionally be satisfied for the time being with a partial solution. The history of success in any art or science is a story of recommencements."*

Systematic thinking, sometimes called the "scientific method" of thinking, can be done by using the five steps of problem-solving. You have probably used these steps before, or at least some of them, but do you know them well enough so that you can use them consciously to solve or prevent problems which you and your staff may encounter?

IDENTIFY AND DEFINE THE PROBLEM.   Perhaps an incident occurs that necessitates action on your part. In many cases the incident itself is not the main problem; rather it is the result of one or more difficulties already existing. It may help you to identify them if you ask yourself, "Why?" or "What?" When you find these underlying causes, you can concentrate on the problem, or several aspects of it, in order to eliminate the major issue.

Some problem areas may be quickly identified by listening to the complaints of your staff. Do they complain about the lack of supplies, difficulty in caring for a certain patient, or the time needed to perform a certain activity, e.g., taking care of doctors' orders?

---

*"In Pursuit of Efficiency." The Royal Bank of Canada Monthly Letter. 50:7:4 (July, 1969).

These complaints usually indicate situations that should be studied and perhaps changed. The complaint itself is not necessarily the real difficulty. Be sure to define the basic problem, not a broad area. Again you must ask the question, "What is happening and why?" In other words, you are ready for the next step.

GET ALL THE FACTS.   Analyze your information to gain as much understanding as possible about the entire situation and its real cause. You may not be able to identify or define the problem completely until you discover these basic issues. Get everyone's version of the incident, or their ideas concerning why the situation exists. Remember that emotions may influence what each person *thinks* she saw or heard. Continue to ask yourself, "Why did this happen?" as well as "What happened?"

Don't jump to a hasty conclusion. Things are not always what they appear to be at first glance. At this point it is important that you keep your thinking as objective as possible. Don't discard an observation because you think that it is contrary to what you *feel* happened. Keep an open mind. Your emotions must be controlled if you are to use the steps of problem-solving effectively. Think of yourself as a detective who considers every clue important to the case being solved.

When you have collected all the available information, sort out that which is essential to your understanding of the problem. Consider each fact by itself, then consider it in relation to the other information you have at hand. Several people may make statements which conflict; therefore, you will need to determine which is most pertinent to the situation you are considering. By this process, you are actually defining the problem. Now you are ready to go on to the next step.

DEVELOP A SOLUTION.   The facts that you have collected should indicate the basic issues in this problem. You must remedy these circumstances if you are to eliminate the situation you first identified as the problem. Ask yourself, "How can I meet this situation? What are the possible results if I handle it in this way?" There are always a number of ways to solve any problem.

You may need to obtain help either from reference reading or from personal interviews. Find out what suggestions others can give. After due consideration, select the suggestion that seems to fit best in your situation.

TAKE ACTION.   Do it now! Don't procrastinate! Decide how to put your solution into effect, then start working. Remember that communicating *what, why,* and *how* is important in gaining the cooperation of your staff. Give everyone a chance to become acquainted with the revised way of doing things. As you talk, stress the advantages of the new method. It is human nature to resist change, but if your coworkers realize how they will benefit, they will be more ready to try.

EVALUATE THE RESULTS. After a trial period, determine your progress. You may not have gained all that you had hoped for, but you should be able to note some improvement. Sometimes a few minor revisions are all that is necessary to make your original plan more effective. Occasionally you may find that your selected method of solving the problem will not work at all. As a leader you cannot afford to scrap the entire project by simply shrugging your shoulders and saying that nothing can be done. Select an alternate solution and work with that for a time; eventually, you will find one that works for you. The important thing is your desire to find a workable solution. You cannot afford to become discouraged; you must continue to have self-confidence and maintain a positive attitude. There is a poem that states in part:

> Success begins with a fellow's will
> It is all in the state of mind.*

That philosophy is very important for a leader in any walk of life.

By using these five steps, you will find that you can handle *any* problem either in a directive or in a creative way. In some problems you will need to gather all the facts, do all the thinking, select what you believe to be the best solution, and inform your staff of the necessary change. By doing this, you are handling the situation in a directive manner. On the other hand, you may help others to recognize the existence of a problem, and then, with their help, develop a plan of action either through discussions with individuals or with your staff as a whole. In this way, you are solving the problem creatively. Often the cooperation of the group is strengthened when the members themselves are allowed to decide on ways of eliminating the circumstances causing the problem.

Illustration in Problem-solving. Imagine that you are having difficulty in getting your staff to report to you about their patients. You feel their failure to report is the problem; however, if you ask yourself *why*, you may find that there are underlying causes, which are the real issues in this situation. Unless you discover these causes, you will never completely gain cooperation in giving the desired reports. Therefore you need to do some investigating.

In this situation, you may work either directively or creatively. In either case, you must search for the answers to the questions, "Does a problem exist?" and "If one exists, what is causing it?" In order to insure patient-centered care, everyone must be kept informed concerning the progress of the patients. Therefore, you are justified in considering your difficulty in obtaining adequate reports

---

*From *The Man Who Thinks He Can.* Anon.

to be a problem. From your personal observation, together with the information given by others, suppose you discover the following facts:

1. Some members of the staff do not always receive enough information about their patients.
2. Some nurses expect to be told only about work that is not finished and nothing personal about the patients.
3. The nurse is not always available to receive this information.
4. Some persons do not know that a report is required of them.
5. Some workers, especially nurses' aides and younger nursing students, do not realize what observations are important and should be reported.

As you analyze these facts and try to understand the entire situation, you realize that a number of underlying issues exist, which cause the situation first identified as the problem. You should also realize that perhaps additional problems are present that you did not recognize in the beginning. In the first place, inconsistencies seem to be present in the methods used to obtain reports from the staff. Also it appears that they do not have a good example to follow. Furthermore, their lack of knowledge predisposes both to their failure to observe well and to their neglect to relay important information, even though they have obtained it.

After due consideration, suppose you decide to define your problem in this way—because all the members of the staff do not always receive a detailed report, they in turn fail to recognize the importance of relaying information. Now ask for suggestions for solving this problem. Perhaps you have some of your own, or you may be able to obtain some ideas from others who have encountered the same situation. Professional journals often contain articles with helpful suggestions for meeting the problems you may encounter in the various aspects of your work.

It is possible that you may obtain the following suggestions:

1. Ask the head nurse to request the staff to tell her—or, if team nursing is used, the team leader—what they have observed about the patients.
2. Discuss the importance of reporting with your group. Include the information you expect their report to contain and help them realize why it is important that you get their report by a certain time.
3. Give a complete report to every person on the staff every day before she begins her work.

4. Always be available to receive reports.
5. Get a report every day even if you have to look up each person to get it.
6. Continue to teach your staff what to observe in various kinds of diseases, and why such observations are important.

Now select the solution or solutions you feel will work best in your situation. Remember to thank and praise each person when she reports to you. Indicate how much her information will help the patient, the doctor and the rest of the staff as they plan the care of the patient. Some may forget occasionally, but give them time and plenty of encouragement. Soon they will learn the value of a good report and if, in addition, you continue to instruct personnel in what to watch for in their patients, you will find the quality of the reports improving also.

In a situation similar to the one used in this illustration, it is entirely inadequate simply to tell the workers that they are required to report. Such a method is extremely dictatorial and will only stimulate resentment toward you and your demands. Lack of understanding is a common reason for failure to follow procedure. You can win their cooperation more quickly by helping them to increase their understanding. Remember that a leader must go ahead and guide; she can never get behind and push.

This is a rather lengthy explanation, and makes it appear that problem-solving is time-consuming. At first, you may find that following through the various steps will take time; however, as you encounter and solve different problems, you will find that it will take less and less time to develop a workable solution because you have more experience and information to guide you.

Management Must Plan a Course of Action. Planning starts with selection of a goal or determining what you hope to accomplish. You will waste time and energy if you fail to have a clear idea of what you want to do. When you know what your destination should be, you will have an easier time deciding how to get there. This means that you must analyze those activities that are essential in providing good care to your patients. You should at the same time try to foresee possible problems and look for some solutions beforehand.

Your aims should define the broad, long-range results of your staff's activities, but you should also set a number of short-term goals which will serve to move the work of the group toward the final objective. Aims must be realistic and reachable in terms of available time, staff, and hospital and community facilities. Policies must be developed to provide guidelines for standards of work performance and patient care. Procedures must also be set up to implement these policies. All policies and procedures must be in writing and must be fully understood by everyone on the staff.

While making your plans, you will be concerned with the various administrative activities already discussed. These include determining what should be done, when, where, how, and who should perform those tasks necessary to accomplish the desired objectives in the most efficient way. The process of efficient work planning will be discussed in the last part of this chapter.

Management Must Organize for Effective Work Performance. Activities must be arranged in workable sequences. Organizing must also include making available the information, equipment, supplies, and other resources that will be needed by the workers. Effective organization requires that the manager delegate responsibility for the performance of the various duties according to job descriptions and the capabilities of the workers. Organizational charts must show the relationships of departments and personnel.

Delegation is an important responsibility of every nurse who is concerned with the management of patient care. When you delegate, you make use of all the functions of management. Here are some suggestions to help you delegate safely and effectively.

1. *Think before you delegate.*   You must decide what you can and what you cannot delegate. You cannot pass along a task or responsibility because it is an unpleasant one or because you do not know what to do. You must also decide to whom you can delegate the selected duties. You cannot delegate tasks or responsibilities that are beyond the ability or the legal right of the individual to perform.

You will want to delegate in order to increase an individual's knowledge and understanding or to help a staff nurse develop her skill in leadership. Routine tasks that do not require judgmental decisions, such as transferring orders, recording information, and ordering supplies, can be delegated after a person has learned the proper procedure to follow.

2. *Be specific when you delegate.* Let people know exactly what they are to do and when. Your directions must be clear, concise, and complete. When delegating a responsibility, you must also give sufficient authority to allow the person to fulfill that responsibility. You must help your staff understand exactly what is expected of them and what they may expect from the other members of the staff. You will need to reinforce the authority you give to others so that everyone recognizes it.

3. *Keep informed after you delegate.* You should get periodic reports from your staff, but you will also want to examine the results of their care by making rounds to all your patients. When something is wrong, discuss it with the person to whom you delegated that

particular responsibility or duty. Also, when the work is well done, you should commend the ones who gave that care.

Management Must Give Directions. Giving directions is one way of carrying out the decisions you made about the delegation of duties and responsibilities to the various members of your staff. Information must be disseminated in such a way that every worker knows exactly what she is to do and how to do it. This entails specific directions, e.g., assignment of patient care; however, it also includes helping the staff understand how they can contribute to the care of every patient, as well as the level of competency expected of each person in her job.

The professional nurse must know her staff well enough to assess them as individuals, what their skills are, and what they need to learn. She must decide whether to use democratic or autocratic leadership as dictated by the needs of the group and the particular situation.

A major aspect of managing involves observation of the activities following the giving of direction. Such observations include continuous scrutiny and evaluation of the work, the workers, their working conditions, and the results of the work performed.

Management Must Exercise Control. Control demands leadership and, whether given autocratically or democratically, causes people to move effectively and cooperatively toward the predetermined goals. It is concerned with the coordination of numerous activities and the making of decisions based upon the planning and organizing activities and the information related to the directing and evaluating of each worker and her performance.

Control in management is concerned with records and reports. These show the progress the organization is making toward achieving its aims and may help to determine where bottlenecks and deficiencies occur. It is also concerned with the most effective use of time, equipment, supplies, and people, for administration is only as effective as the people who make up the entire organization help it to be.

The techniques of planning, organizing, directing, and controlling are necessary components of the process called supervision; consequently, both management and supervision help administration achieve its aims.

METHODS OF WORK IMPROVEMENT

Sometimes hospital administrators ask industrial engineers to review the activities on the nursing units and to make suggestions for more efficient work methods. Because this person is often machine-oriented, he may emphasize those procedures which are related to the production of tangible results which may be reached at a calculated speed, e.g., the number of baths given or beds made, while giving little attention to the recipient of these ministrations, the patient.

Often this person views nursing as consisting only of manual skills or techniques of varying complexity; consequently, he fails to realize that in nursing we are working with unpredictable machines, i.e., the patient as well as the worker; and that we are concerned with an intangible product, i.e., nursing care that cannot be standardized on the basis of quantity per hour. If our primary concern is for the patient, we may have to take longer to give him a bath today than we did yesterday. However, through the application of work improvement methods, we can find ways of performing those nursing techniques and activities more efficiently.

The purpose of this discussion is to introduce the reader to the main fundamentals of work improvement. Those who wish to acquire a greater understanding of the subject should read the books and articles listed in the bibliography or, better yet, take a course in time and motion study or work simplification.

Purpose of Work Improvement Studies. These studies consist of an organized approach to a situation in order to solve work problems. At times people feel that the analysis and changing of existing routines and procedures is done so that the administration can require them to do more work. This is not true; however, this belief must be changed if the proposed alterations are to be accepted by the staff. When people do not accept given reasons for change, they will sabotage any new method, either consciously or unconsciously.

What then are the reasons for using these methods of work improvement or work simplification in your job?

To MAKE A PERSON'S WORK EASIER AND SAFER. The worker will be able to get just as much done but with less effort and with greater safety for herself, her coworkers, and her patients. We all use shortcuts which we find accidentally or observe others using. Such shortcuts are not always safe. Work improvement methods provide a systematic way for determining shortcuts without affecting the quality of our work.

To ELIMINATE WASTE OF TIME AND SUPPLIES. Time and supplies cost money, which eventually comes from a patient because of higher costs for patient care. We should devise techniques that take less time to do or that use less expensive equipment or less equipment. When analyzing our activities, we must consider not only the equipment we use but also the time and cost necessary for its maintenance. We must also analyze the time we use to perform a procedure, e.g., put on hot packs or transcribe doctors' orders onto the Kardex.

To ELIMINATE DUPLICATION OF PERSONNEL OR EFFORT. Time also enters into this purpose. Sometimes a study shows that two or even three people are performing the same function. With some revisions the work can be done by one person, thus allowing others more time to perform their other duties. Very often one individual is performing the same activity several times when the same result could be reached in a single effort, e.g., making a single trip to the laundry chute to dispose of used linens from several patients instead of carrying them to the chute after the care of each patient. Elimination of duplication may aid in safety for the patients because it decreases the chance for errors of both omission and commission.

To IMPROVE PATIENT CARE. When the previous reasons for work simplification are accepted and the suggestions implemented, the end result will be improvement in efficiency and effectiveness in giving patient care. When we find more efficient ways for giving care and for managing the unit, we will have more time and opportunity to give the kind of care we say we want to give our patients.

The repeated excuse, "... but I don't have the time," is frequently no longer valid. Thomas Edison had a motto above his desk which read, "There is a better way. Find it." If we would approach our various duties and responsibilities in a systematic way, we would be able to find many ways of saving time, allowing us that time we think we need to give better patient care.

How to Solve Work Problems. Applying the principles of work improvement makes use of the same steps that are used in problem-solving. Fredrick W. Taylor* first proposed the use of systematic studies in industry which he called scientific management. Frank and Lillian Gilbreth** initiated methods of analyzing work through motion-study techniques in order to eliminate all unnecessary movements by the worker, decreasing fatigue yet maintaining or improving his work output.

STEP 1. SELECT A PROBLEM. Selecting a problem is not always easy. Questions frequently asked are: What kind of problem? Should it be concerned with nursing care or with a procedure? How do we recognize a problem?

A problem exists when any activity can be performed more efficiently or effectively than it is now being done. A problem area may be found by listening to the complaints of patients or their families, or of the staff. Sometimes we do not recognize a problem because we either do not look for one or do not question or study what we see and hear. In the management of patient care the nurse must be alert for indications of problem areas. Uncompleted work, work delays or interruptions, or taking too long to complete a specif-

---

*Taylor, Fredrick Winslow: *Scientific Management.* Harper and Row, 1947.
**Gilbreth, Frank: *Motion Study.* Van Nostrand-Reinhold, New York, 1911.

ic job may be indications that more efficient methods should be looked for. Excessive turnover in staff should be studied to determine causes and, if possible, remedied. Errors in carrying out assigned duties and responsibilities must always be studied to determine their cause and prevention. High costs resulting from loss or damage of equipment and waste of supplies are always indications that poor management exists.

Other general areas on a nursing unit in which problems may exist include:

1. Administrative or managerial activities
    Supervision of various levels of the staff
    Revising policy and procedure manuals
    Revising job descriptions
2. Clerical activities
    Delivering telephone messages to patients
    Ordering supplies
    Charting information on patients' charts
3. Housekeeping activities
    Cleaning units following patient discharges
    Distributing and collecting linen
    Caring for flowers
4. Dietary activities
    Filling out daily menus
    Serving patient trays
5. Techniques used in patient care
    Nursing care planning conferences
    Administration of medicines
    Getting patients up, e.g., into wheelchairs or on crutches
6. Physical lay-out of the station and the use of supplies, space, and time spent in non-nursing activities
    Place for storage of stretcher
    Storage of supplies compared to place of use
    Disposal of used equipment or linen
7. Interdepartmental activities or relationships
    Delivering reports, schedules, and requisitions
    Scheduling times for physical therapy or x-ray activities
    Time for serving meals to patients
    Moving patients from one department to another

With a little thought you should be able to find examples of situations on your unit in which improvement is needed. Perhaps you may want to use different classifications for the general areas.

When you have finally selected what you want to study, be sure that you have isolated a single problem. Sometimes we find what we think is one problem, only to find that it consists of a number of problems which may be interrelated but sometimes are entirely unrelated. Divide each of the problems into as many parts as possible. Study first the situations that are the easiest to learn about; then proceed to the more complex. Be sure that no part of an individual problem, no step in the procedure, is omitted.

STEP 2. STUDY THE PROBLEM.   Get as much information as possible about the situation selected for study. Methods for gathering facts include job analysis or activity analysis, work flow graphs, work distribution charts, and others. These are somewhat technical, though not difficult, methods and will not be discussed in great detail in this book. Those who are interested may do additional study by consulting the bibliography.

When the facts have been listed, they may be studied by using Kipling's "six honest serving men"—What, Why, When, Where, How, and Who. A simple method which can be used quite effectively if people really are anxious to find better ways of doing their jobs uses these same questions and is sometimes called the Planning Formula.

1. *What?* What should be done? What was done? What equipment and supplies? What time is needed? What steps in the procedure? What sequence of activities was used? What other method could be used?
2. *When?* When should the job be done? When was it done? When could it be done?
3. *Where?* Where is the job done? Where does activity occur in relation to activities immediately preceding and following? Where else could supplies be stored, cleaned, and so forth?
4. *How?* How is the job done, i.e., what are the steps in the procedure? How are the time and energy of personnel being used throughout?
5. *Who?* Who is doing the job? Who else could do it? Is more than one person involved?
6. *Why?* To each of the above questions, ask *Why.* Why is this job, this procedure, this step necessary? Why is it done in this way, in this place, at this time, by this person?

You will note that all the questions are concerned with procedures and activities. At this time we are not thinking of the physical and mental activities which the professional nurse uses to plan the nursing care and, to a certain extent, to give that care to her patients.

You may approach the study of work problems in several different ways.

1. Determine what activities are performed by each level of worker. This may be done by an observer listing at 15 minutes intervals what each person is doing. Staff personnel may record their own activities and the time used. These

studies should cover several days in order to get a good
sampling of activities and time.

2. Determine what personnel perform predetermined activities.
   An observer should record how many times the head nurse —
   or the staff nurse, or L.P.N., or a nursing aid, or the ward
   secretary — answers the telephone.

3. Determine the total time spent in each of a number of selected activities during a specified time. For example, how
   much time does the head nurse use to check charts, make out
   medication cards, or make out condition or other reports?

4. Analyze steps and movements in a specific procedure. This
   analysis can be done best by using work flow diagrams and
   work analysis charts, also called flow process charts. These
   two techniques of study are described here in more detail.

Work Flow Diagram.   The work flow diagram is a simple way of
studying the movements necessary to complete a certain job. It can
be used alone or with the flow process chart. A flow diagram may
describe an activity on a single unit or one which moves from one
department to another.

Steps in making a work flow diagram are:

1. Prepare a scale drawing of the work area including furniture,
   doors, partitions, and any other features normally used in
   completing the job.

2. Indicate by a line the usual path and direction the worker
   uses to perform the activity being studied.

3. Insert important information, e.g., what is done at various
   locations, time, and distance covered.

To illustrate this technique a simple work flow diagram shows a
method used in one hospital to dispose of used linens (Fig. 2).

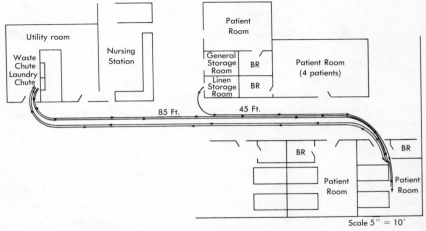

Figure 2.   Present method of used linen disposal.

WORK ANALYSIS CHART

Job _Disposal of used linen_
Activity Studied _disposal of used linens from 2 patients_
Job Begins _Bath pack in the storage room_
Job Ends _Disposal bag placed in laundry chute_
Suggestions _Use hamper to collect linen from several patients_

Date ___3-10-70___

Summary	Totals
O--Operation	12
T--Transportation	4
I--Inspection	0
D--Delay	2
S--Storage	1
Total distance	300 feet
Total time	hours 3/4 minutes

#	Description of Motion	O	T	I	D	S	FEET	TIME	Notes
1	Nurse gets bath pack from linen room					●			Linen disposal bag is in bath pack
2	Takes pack to patient's room		/				45	30 sec.	
3	Removes used top linens from bed of patient A	/							
4	Places used linens on chair	●							
5	Used linens wait on chair				\				
6	Removes rest of used linens when bottom of bed is made up	/							
7	Places all soiled linen in bag	●							
8	Closes bag with draw string	●							
9	Takes bag to utility room		\				85	55 sec.	
10	Places bag in laundry chute	<							
11	Nurse returns to patient's room		\				85	55 sec.	
12	Removes used top linens from bed of patient B.	/							
13	Places used linens on chair	●							
14	Used linens wait on chair				\				
15	Removes rest of used linens when making up bottom of bed	/							
16	Places all soiled linen in disposal bag	●							
17	Closes bag with draw string	●							
18	Takes bag to utility room		\				85	55 sec.	
19	Places bag in laundry chute	/							
20				Totals			300 ft	195 sec. ÷ 60 = 3/4 min.	
21									
22									
23									
24									
25									

Figure 3. Disposal of used linen.

Work Analysis or Flow Process Chart. Printed forms used by industrial engineers may be obtained for this type of study; however, you may develop a very simple form for your own use as illustrated in Figure 3.

The process chart records the step-by-step movements of a job. It analyzes a series of motions indicating the result achieved in each step. These results are described as follows:

1. *Operation:* When something is added or changed.
2. *Transportation:* When a person or material moves from one place to another.
3. *Inspection:* When something is looked at, checked, but not changed.
4. *Delay:* When a person or material is waiting or activity is interrupted.

5. *Storage:* When something stays in one place awaiting action.

In recording events on the work analysis chart, the observer must identify the specific activity being studied. She should also show at what point the analysis starts and where it ends. Each job must be carefully separated into individual steps or motions. The total results should be summarized including total motion or distance travelled and time involved.

STEP 3. DEVISE A NEW METHOD. In finding a different and better way of doing our work, we may eliminate some things that we have been doing, rearrange the sequence or combine two or more activities, or perhaps find an entirely new method in order to simplify our work, making it easier and more efficient.

The questions *What* and *Why* will help to determine which activities are necessary, and to establish priorities. They will also indicate bottlenecks and the reasons for errors. The answers may lead to the elimination of those activities or steps which do not help in reaching the objectives of the particular job.

The questions *Where, When, Who,* and *How* will give you ideas about how to combine activities, rearrange the steps in a more effective sequence, or simplify an activity. Sometimes you will find that you can accomplish more by adding one or two steps or rearranging the steps in an existing procedure, rather than devising an entirely new procedure.

STEP 4. PUTTING THE NEW METHOD TO WORK. To do something in a different way means that change must occur. We must accept the fact that change is normal and that without change no progress can be made. Accepting changes and new ideas is not only a manager's responsibility in leadership; it is also the responsibility of each worker.

Getting people to accept change is largely a matter of "selling" the idea. Getting new ideas to work effectively is one of the biggest tests of the abilities of a supervisor, head nurse, or staff nurse who wants to be a leader. In order to sell an idea, she must know the individuals on her staff well enough to understand the roadblocks which they may erect to keep it from working. She must understand people well enough to select the best arguments and the best methods to persuade them to accept and try a new idea.

OBSTACLES TO CHANGE

Emotions.   One of the biggest obstacles to change comes from emotional blocks—our own and others'. When we are sold on an idea, we become *impatient* and want to see the proposed change take place immediately. One of the quickest ways of killing a good idea is to force people to accept it.

A bit of doggerel by an unknown author states:

"A man convinced against his will
Is of the same opinion still."

Another emotional obstacle is *fear*—our own and others'. It is human nature to relate everything that happens to ourselves. When a change is proposed, each person will immediately ask, "How will this affect me and my job?" Change is threatening to the security of the individual. Different people will see different meanings or threats in any proposed change, and a feeling of anxiety or fear develops—fear of job insecurity, fear of learning new techniques, fear of being required to produce more work, either quantitatively or qualitatively. Underneath all these fears lies the basic fear of failure, of not being able to function acceptably in the new situation. However, people do not want to admit that they are afraid so they offer various excuses or display various attitudes of resistance which they think will be more socially acceptable.

THE "IT WON'T WORK" OR "I HAVEN'T TIME" ATTITUDE. These are the most common excuses offered for not trying something different. People use them whenever they are faced with a demand for change when they do not want to change. If they are forced to accept the new method against their wishes, they will do everything in their power to make it fail and, whenever possible, revert to the old way again. Under such conditions, any new plan is bound to fail, and when it does, the personnel will quickly adopt the "see, I told you" attitude. When this is allowed to happen, any future changes will be extremely difficult to make.

Habits. People are creatures of habit and always tend to drift back to an old, and for them comfortable, rut. Changes and new ideas require thought and exertion to break old habits. Most people dislike to be forced to think. When starting something different, people must be allowed to participate in the development of new ideas and have an opportunity to become acquainted with them.

One of the habits which are most difficult to break is the habit of criticism. It is always easier to see what is wrong with a new idea or technique than to see the benefits to be derived from accepting it. People must be helped to see how they will benefit, i.e., how it will help them learn more, make their work easier, improve their job status or feeling of self-worth, or help them give better patient care.

Self-satisfaction. One of the greatest hindrances to progress is the inability of people to see any need for improvement, either as individuals or as a group. "Our patients get good care" is a comment offered by hospital personnel who fail to realize that their statement in itself proves that they should not be so self-satisfied. *Good* implies various degrees of performance, with the degrees of *better* and *best* not being attained, according to their own evaluation.

No change will occur until people become dissatisfied with themselves and the way they are doing something. This feeling of dissatisfaction then provides the stimulus to make them want to try something different.

GETTING THE DESIRED RESPONSES

Select Practical and Reachable Goals.   Establish priorities – do first things first. Concentrate on one or two areas where a change will show outstanding results. A feeling of success makes it easier for everyone to try something else.

Keep Everyone Informed.   Tell them about the proposed changes and the reasons for them. Be honest. Give them all the facts. Let them know these changes will affect them and what will be expected of them.

Get Them Involved.   Give them a chance to offer suggestions. Give credit when their suggestions are practical. Show that you have faith in their ability to solve problems, and then they will try to meet your expectations. Pittsburgh's PPG Industries brought small groups of employees together in "value analysis sessions." These employees suggested ways of saving $200,000 a year by cutting down on the paper work.* The more chances that people have to participate in deciding about changes, the harder they will try to make their ideas work.

Keep Your Eyes on the Desired Goal but Remember That There Are Many Ways of Getting There.   Perhaps someone will suggest a better way than the one you originally thought of. You too must be willing to change when necessary.

SIX SUGGESTIONS TO HELP YOU SAVE TIME

1. Determine What You Want to Accomplish.   A lot of people waste time and energy because they do not know what they want to do. Ask youself, "What must be done? What must I do?" Maybe you have to write a report, give an 8 o'clock medication, find ways to get a patient to exercise her arm, or determine why a nurses' aide is unable to finish her assignment. Whatever it is, define it clearly in your mind.

2. Establish Priorities.   Do the „most important things first. One executive challenged efficiency expert Ivy Lee to show him how to get things done when they had to be done. This was Lee's advice.

---

*Time, Feb. 16, 1970, p. 79.

List in order of their importance the most urgent jobs you must do. Tomorrow morning start in on the first one and stick with it until you finish it. Then go to the second one and finish it, and so on. Do not worry if you finish only two or three by the end of the day, because you will be concentrating on the most important ones. If your work cannot be done by this method, you cannot complete it by any other method. A month later the executive sent Lee a check for $25,000 and a letter of thanks for the "most profitable lesson" of his life.

While you may not be able to carry out this suggestion in exactly this way, you can get more done if you establish priorities. The secret of those people who seem to get so much done is that they put first things first. A big job can be finished quickly and more easily if you take one step at a time. Get into the habit of making notes. Even top executives keep appointment calendars to remind themselves of important activities. The paper and pencil habit can save you time by refreshing your memory about important information and duties.

Perhaps you cannot get things done because you are trying to do too much. Establishing priorities requires delegation. You must determine what you yourself must do and what you can give to someone else.

3. Have Respect for Your Own Time and for That of Others. If you earn $7000 a year plus various benefits such as paid vacation and sick time, your time is worth approximately $5\frac{1}{2}$ cents a minute. At $9000 a year your time is worth about 8 cents a minute. Putting a monetary value on time may help you gain a new respect for it, especially when you waste it.

Don't waste the time of others. Their time is valuable too. Recurrent crises can usually be foreseen and prevented. Anticipate your own needs and those of your staff. Have all the necessary supplies on hand before they must be used. Help your staff use their time and energies efficiently.

Listen to questions, instructions, and reports. Getting all the information right the first time will save time and prevent costly and sometimes dangerous errors. If you need additional information, you should ask questions and get answers immediately. Answering a worker's questions promptly will save you time later on and perhaps keep her from making a mistake.

Be sure that everyone has all the information needed, given at one time. An excess of meetings wastes time. One either meets or one works. When everyone knows all that he needs to know to do his job satisfactorily and has the necessary materials available, there is no need for repeated meetings. This does not mean that they will not want help. Help and guidance may be greatly needed during the performance of the work.

4. Do It Now.   If you have something that must be done, get started on it immediately and keep with it until you finish it. Sharpening your pencil, gazing out the window, having a cup of coffee, doing something else first are all time-wasters. It may be human nature to procrastinate, but it is certainly unproductive.

5. Establish Deadlines.   Commit yourself to a schedule, but make it realistic. Stick to your schedule to avoid procrastination. When you meet your deadline, reward yourself with something you really want—a new dress, a trip, reading a book, a coffee break. Deny yourself this reward if you fail to meet your schedule on time. Be as firm with yourself as you would be with a member of your staff who must get something done by a certain time.

6. Keep Looking for More Efficient Ways of Doing Your Work.   With a little more knowledge, understanding, and thought almost any activity can be streamlined without detracting from the quality of the end result. How about delegating some additional duties to the ward secretary? How can you save time by using a tape recorder? Perhaps a different sequence of assignments will save time. Are you really accomplishing something when you do it this way? In other words, take a good look at your job and apply the principles of work simplification. You might be surprised at the time you could save.

Leadership is the key to effective management. Nursing leadership in management of patient care provides the motivation and guidance which help the nursing staff achieve their goal of improving patient care.

STUDY QUESTIONS

1. Select several policies of your institution and trace the way they are implemented in specific procedures.

2. List at least five principles to be observed when delegating duties and responsibilities.

3. Identify at least four work problems on your unit. Study each problem, using a different method of analysis if at all possible. For each problem suggest a way of improving the method presently in use or devise a new method.

4. What techniques did you use to devise this new method?

5. Discuss how you would implement your suggestions for change in Question 3 above. Be sure to consider possible cost or saving to the institution or patient, probable results in patient care, people affected and so forth.

6. Analyze your own work and suggest ten specific ways by which you can save time and energy. How will you use the time that you save?

Chapter 6

Leadership in Nursing

Administration and supervision are correlative, and the effectiveness of each depends upon the quality of leadership given to it. It seems impossible to divide these subjects into three, or even two, separate entities; rather, when one is being considered, its relation to the other must also be considered. Sometimes nursing administration, nursing supervision, and nursing leadership are spoken of as though they were three different areas of nursing endeavor or responsibility. Perhaps it would be better to think of them as interrelated activities that are part of the duties of every professional nurse.

YOUR TYPE OF LEADERSHIP – DIRECTIVE OR CREATIVE?

Your method of leadership will vary according to the existing situation and may change from day to day, even from hour to hour. People will be watching you, listening to you, deciding how they feel about you. Their decision will be based upon your ability to put your leadership across. If they feel ignored, not part of the in-group, or necessary only to get the work done, you may find yourself a leader in name only.

Suppose that one morning you are assigned a new and inexperienced aide. Remember that first impressions are often lasting impressions. It is important that your leadership start from the moment she becomes a part of your group. You must make her feel that she is needed, for with that feeling comes the desire to participate and cooperate in the unit's activities. Introducing yourself and the other members of the group is important. It is also important that she recognize that you are the one to whom she can come for help. You will probably want to use directive leadership at first, since she is new in the hospital situation and is likely to be unsure of herself. Make sure that she understands her duties—what she is to do, when, and how; to whom she is to report, and why. It is never wise to allow another worker of the same rank to be responsible for this period of orientation.

An emergency arises—a patient's condition suddenly becomes critical, an accident case is admitted in the middle of a busy morning. Your staff will look to you for instructions about what to do; again you will use directive leadership. Decisions must be made immediately —what to do, how to do it, and who is best qualified. Everyone works together, but you give specific directions. You are the leader—the one who knows the way. Yet when the emergency is past, you did not meet it alone; you and your coworkers met it together. This is the result of leadership. Remember to give credit for cooperation and for a job done well together.

These are only two examples of situations in which you will find that directive leadership is necessary; there will be others. In each case you will use the method of leadership that best meets the needs of your staff and the needs of your patients.

As you gain experience, your leadership can become more democratic or creative. You should recognize the contribution that each person is capable of making toward meeting the needs of the patients, and you should encourage each person to obtain a greater understanding of nursing care. As people gain this understanding, you should give them more opportunities to suggest ways of meeting various patient care problems, rather than telling them how. You should encourage each one to participate in the planning of patient care. This does not mean that your leadership will become less. Actually, your leadership should become greater than before, for you must continually seek ways in which you and your staff can improve the care of your patients. Remember that the quality of patient care, the quality of team play, the quality of respect for each person as an individual will be no greater than those which you demonstrate in your leadership. These concepts provide the challenge of creative leadership in nursing.

TECHNIQUES IN LEADERSHIP IN NURSING

You must be aware of and willing to accept the responsibilities of leadership. You must know each person, recognizing each one's needs and differences as individuals. You must be able to help each one satisfy her needs. You will need to make allowances for her different abilities, attitudes, feelings and emotions. In other words,

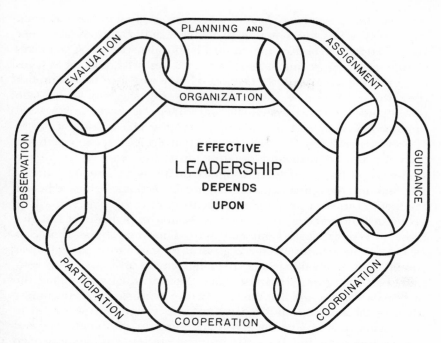

PLANNING AND
EVALUATION
ASSIGNMENT
ORGANIZATION
OBSERVATION
EFFECTIVE
LEADERSHIP
DEPENDS
UPON
GUIDANCE
PARTICIPATION
COOPERATION
COORDINATION

Figure 4. Leadership is only as strong as the weakest link in this chain.

you must give your staff a "psychological paycheck." You must understand the principles and techniques employed in administration and supervision, as well as those employed in giving patient care, for your leadership must be guided by these principles and techniques. For example, you may not be concerned with making out hours for the staff on the station, but you will be, or should be, concerned with making the best use of their time and energy. If you have a unit manager, you may not be concerned with the ordering of supplies for use by the entire station, but you will certainly be concerned about seeing that the supplies are not wasted.

Planning and Organizing.   Plan and organize your own work. Coordinate all activities so that everything gets done at the proper time and in the correct way. Perhaps you have had the unhappy experience of working with a person who "flits" from one job to another; makes frequent trips to get equipment and supplies, which she forgot to bring with her the first time; neglects to remind someone to do something until it is too late; works too fast; talks too fast; and looks hurried and breathless. Soon those who work with her look and act the same way. The patients feel the pressure and, although they may not realize exactly why, they are not comfortable or relaxed. These are the results of disorganization.

On the other hand, you may know a nurse who, when an emergency arises, does not seem to move any faster or raise her voice. People can be rushing around frantically, yet, when she takes charge, everyone seems to relax. Order is restored, and the work is done quickly in an orderly fashion. How is she able to accomplish this? Does she possess some magic? No, but she is a leader who thinks and acts in a systematic way. There is never any wasted motion. She knows what to do and the most efficient way to do it. However, she did not acquire this ability overnight. It came with her learning how to plan and organize, first, her work as a nursing student, and later, her more complex duties as a graduate nurse.

Making Assignments and Giving Directions. Regardless of the method used in making assignments in your hospital, you will be giving directions; therefore, you must be able to plan ahead and give those directions clearly and concisely. They may be as simple as asking a nurses' aide to take a glassful of water to a patient or as complicated as making and explaining patient assignments to your staff. In either case, you must make the individual understand the directions you are giving. You are also responsible for determining whether the task is completed in the proper way. You will need to work with people who have varying degrees of experience and knowledge, from the freshman nursing student or inexperienced nurses' aide to the experienced practical nurse or even the professional nurse. You will need to use all your knowledge and understanding of human relations and nursing techniques.

Guidance. Guidance is a valuable tool in the hands of the nurse. The word *guidance* implies going before, leading the way, and makes use of various teaching and counseling methods. In addition to having a thorough knowledge of nursing and its many skills, you must have the ability to help each member of your staff perform her assigned duties both to her own satisfaction and to the satisfaction of the patient.

This does not mean that you will become a counselor in the usual sense of the word. It does, however, mean that you must recognize the relationship of personal problems and emotions to the ability of the individual to do a good job. It also means that, by example, you will demonstrate what you expect of each person in giving nursing care and understanding to the patient.

Cooperation. You must cooperate with and encourage cooperation among your coworkers. Leadership is essential if you are to have teamwork. The amount of cooperation that exists will depend greatly upon you and your attitude toward them as individuals. Remember that they are working *with* you, not *for* or *under* you. The idea of subservience, indicated by the words *for* and *under*, implies extreme directive leadership and stifles the feeling of cooperation essential to the effective care of patients.

Cooperation is encouraged by an atmosphere of democracy in which the individual knows what is expected of her, is kept informed of her progress, and is stimulated to improve through the praise and constructive criticism skillfully given by the leader. Let your staff know that you have confidence in them. Do not ask them to do something which you would not be willing to do yourself. Say "will you" more often than "you must." Good human relations stimulate cooperation and loyalty.

Encouraging Participation. You should provide opportunities for the participation of each person in the activities of the unit. Working with a group fosters the feeling of belonging to that group. Participation may take various forms, depending upon the person's abilities and desires. It does not imply merely talking at team conferences or doing a certain amount of work, although these are certainly desirable forms of participation. Cooperation is closely allied to participation; both must be active rather than passive.

You will need to provide obvious opportunities for the cooperation and participation by the individual who tends to be withdrawn and passive. Recognition for her participation is important to her. Even though she may be wrong—for example, giving information that is incomplete or incorrect during a discussion—you should recognize her contribution, although you will need to correct her.

Coordination. Coordination of activities within the unit is a necessary part of nursing leadership. You need to keep everyone informed about the various ward and hospital activities. Also you need to report to your immediate superior about the work accomplished by your staff. You will want to utilize the services of other people or agencies, thereby making all of the hospital and community resources available to the patient. You will need to plan to prevent conflicts in the performance of duties as your staff go about their work. Coordination is based upon good planning and the utilization of the abilities of each person and the resources found within the hospital and surrounding community.

Observation. The observation of your staff and their work is one of your biggest responsibilities. Observation must be more than just checking and inspecting; it is the acquisition of knowledge through the use of all of your senses. You need to be able to see patient care in its entirety as well as its individual aspects. To do this you will need to observe not only the physical performance of the worker but also the manifestations of those abstract areas involving her emotions and understanding.

Evaluation. Not only must you learn to observe correctly, but you must also learn to evaluate your observations. Evaluation should be a continuous process of analyzing the strengths and the weaknesses that you observe in the personnel themselves or in their work, so that you can encourage them to continue doing good work or help them to improve in those areas in which they are weak. To be able to analyze fairly, you must set up some definite goals beforehand and have direct personal contact with the persons and the work you want to evaluate; otherwise, you have nothing on which you can base your judgment.

You must also evaluate yourself, as a person, as a nurse, and as a leader; for, if you are unable to criticize yourself honestly, you have no right to criticize others. This ability to do self-evaluation is one of the attributes that every leader must develop.

But after evaluation, what? Is your work finished? By no means! After determining the effectiveness of patient care on your unit, and where you need to improve, you will need to set new goals, make new plans, reorganize your resources, and begin work again. Leadership can never become static; for, when it rests on past achievements, there is no longer any leadership.

DO YOU HAVE WHAT IT TAKES TO BE A LEADER?

Qualities Needed by a Leader. A leader must possess certain definite qualities. First of all, she must be a professional nurse in every sense of the word. She must be willing to assume those responsibilities concomitant with her profession. Not only must she know what constitutes good nursing care but also she must give good care to her patients. She must be interested in people and be able to communicate with them effectively.

Good health is very necessary, for it is closely related to emotions and influences, to a great extent, how the nurse feels about her work and toward those with whom she is working.

A leader must also be a follower. This may sound contradictory, yet the democratic leader helps her group decide what should be done and is guided by their suggestions. In nursing especially, there must be united effort and a constant interchange of ideas.

One of the most important qualities for a leader is emotional maturity. This kind of maturity has nothing to do with physical age; rather, it implies that the individual has reached a stage in her development when she has become independent in thought and action, with the ability to make decisions based on her analysis of all available facts. The mature person is more concerned with others than with herself; she thinks more about giving than getting. She does not dwell on the past and its errors, although she uses the lessons learned through them to improve herself. She has learned to criticize herself objectively and is flexible enough to try to change those personal characteristics that she feels are not consistent with what she wants to be. She has also learned that she is only human and, therefore, not perfect; consequently, she tries to be tolerant of others, abhorring the faults but not the individual. She strives to be consistent and fair in all her dealings.

Leadership is not free; it demands the price of great mental and physical effort, of more self-criticism, self-control, and self-confidence. In fact, Eleanor C. Lambertsen* maintains that "a primary factor in successful leadership is the leader's belief in the philosophy of the nursing team, and in the confidence she feels in her ability as a leader."

WHAT KIND OF LEADER DOES YOUR STAFF WANT?

When talking with nursing assistants and L.P.N.'s, I always ask for their suggestions as to how the registered nurses can help them. The suggestions given most often by these people include:

1. Giving a report about *all* the patients before we start our patient care.
2. Giving an explanation of our assignment—*how* to care for our patients, not just a check list of things to be done telling only *what* and *when*.
3. *Showing* us how to give the care to a patient instead of just *telling* us the steps of a procedure.
4. *Listening* to us when we report and checking our patients when we ask the R.N. to look at them.

Time and again a nursing aide tells how afraid she felt when assigned to care for a critically ill or dying patient and how much she wanted someone to come and help her. The help these people are asking for is more than physical assistance; it is help in meeting an unfamiliar, frightening experience. They want someone who is unafraid because she knows what to do and how to do it skillfully and who is willing to pass on this knowledge to them. Are you meeting their needs?

DECALOGUE FOR LEADERSHIP

1. Thou Shalt Seek Continually After Knowledge and Strive to Attain Understanding and Wisdom. Knowledge, understanding, and wisdom are not synonymous. The professional nurse must be a

---

*Lambertsen, Eleanor C.: *Nursing Team—Organization and Functioning.* Published for the Division of Nursing Education by the Bureau of Publications, Teachers College, Columbia, 1953, page 22.

continual learner not only of new methods and skills but also of new ideas and concepts in nursing. Yet knowledge of facts and concepts, or even of methods, is of no value unless it is combined with *understanding*, i.e., the ability to see relationships. Understanding includes the ability to take different ideas and bits of information and fit them together in a meaningful way so that they may be used in the care of a patient. *Wisdom* goes a step further and implies the ability to select the best idea or the best method for a particular patient or situation. Wisdom cannot be taught although methods of evaluation on which wisdom is based can be learned. Wisdom comes with making good use of all experiences in the clinical area, in the classroom, in family and social situations, in everyday living.

2. Thou Shalt Set a Goal and Continue to Strive to Reach it. The nurse must know where she wants to go and must set up guidelines to help herself get there. This means setting personal goals—what kind of person does she want to become? It means setting professional goals—what kind of nurse does she want to become? It means setting nursing goals—what can she do for her patient or help him do for himself? Such goals must be broad, long-term, looking toward the future; however, there must be more specific, short-term goals to help her know how near she is to her main goal. The concept can best be expressed as a state of *becoming* rather than of *being** because main goals should be far enough beyond reach so there is always something to look toward. This thought is implied in the quotation from the Sanskrit, "Tomorrow is always a vision of hope. Look well therefore to this day!"

3. Thou Shalt Be Able and Willing to Accept Responsibility. Acceptance of responsibility is the essence of nursing leadership. It requires the use of professional knowledge, understanding, and wisdom to set up appropriate goals, the willingness to use one's judgment, to make decisions, and then to put those decisions into action. Willingness to accept responsibility for one's own actions is a characteristic of any leader. Willingness to accept the responsibility necessary in the guidance and supervision of other personnel is required of the nurse who wishes to function as a professional nursing practitioner. A nursing leader cannot think that she is better than any of her followers except in the degree of her acceptance of responsibility.

4. Thou Shalt Develop Initiative and Enthusiasm. At first glance these two qualities may appear to be entirely unrelated, but this is not true. Initiative, the ability to recognize what should be done and to go ahead and do it, is closely related to enthusiasm,

*Maslow, A. H.: *Toward a Psychology of Being*. Van Nostrand, Princeton, New Jersey, 1962, Chapt. 5.

which implies interest in getting the thing done. The opposite of enthusiasm is boredom, and a bored person rarely exerts enough energy to do his work well, let alone look for additional ways to improve in his job. Enthusiasm makes the difference between living and just existing. It puts something into life. It is thinking positively. Enthusiasm can lead to success and happiness as a person, as a nurse, as a leader.

5. Thou Shalt Not Lose Thy Sense of Humor. Some years ago the finalists in a beauty contest were asked to name "the greatest man in the world" and to tell why. Some chose famous scientists, statesmen, or humanitarians. But one girl said without hesitation, "Bob Hope. He makes the world laugh by laughing at himself!"

Do not take yourself too seriously. Learn to see yourself as others see you; then smile at what you see. Laughter is a great gift and is needed in our daily lives. Laughing at yourself can make life pleasanter for yourself and others, and it can also take the sting out of unpleasant situations when used correctly. Learn to laugh *with* but never *at* other people. Laugh only at yourself. A well-known psychiatrist once said that he had never had to treat anyone who could really laugh at himself. Laughter is an ointment that smooths away the tensions and irritations of a hectic day.

6. Thou Shalt Strive to Give a "Psychological Paycheck" to Those with Whom You Work. Even in this materialistic age money is not everything. We are sometimes so concerned with our patients and their needs that we neglect our coworkers and their needs and feelings. They want to know what is going on, to be appreciated, not only as a person but also as a coworker in the giving of patient care. Sometimes the biggest "paycheck" is given when the nurse says, "Thank you. You did a good job," and her coworker knows she really means it.

7. Thou Shalt Be More Interested in Others Than in Thyself. Sometimes a nurse will manipulate others so they satisfy her needs instead of her trying to satisfy theirs. The nurse who wants to be needed, to be important to someone, may try to keep others dependent upon her when they should be learning to think for themselves. If she feels insecure, she will seek constant reassurance from those around her, never giving a thought that they may need reassurance too. When a person becomes too concerned about her own feelings, she will be unable to function as a leader because a leader must be emotionally stable and mature enough to understand herself and be comfortable with herself before she can be comfortable working with other people. She must be more interested in how she can help them than in what she can get from them.

8. Thou Shalt Not Be Too Quick to Judge Others. Jumping to conclusions usually means that prejudice has influenced your judgment. Be fair. Get all the facts and verify each one. The evaluation of a person cannot be made on one instance of behavior. There may be times when the nurse should not judge at all. At times one should accept the person as he is, listen to him, and recognize his right to have positive and negative feelings.

9. Thou Shalt Not Lose Thy Self-control. When a person loses control of himself, he also loses control of the situation. Anger prevents a person from thinking clearly. Unless the safety of a person is involved, the nurse should never do or say anything until she is over her anger. She should never react with anger to anger in another person. This ability to control herself takes a great amount of understanding of people and how they act. Self-control will make you the master — a leader — in any situation.

10. Thou Shalt Not Become Self-satisfied. When we become self-satisfied, we stagnate. This is one of the big problems in nursing today. We are trying to practice nursing in the 1970's using the same methods, attitudes, and concepts that we used ten, twenty, or even thirty years ago. We seek to justify our practice by saying, "This is the way that has always worked for us. Those newfangled notions just won't work on my station, in our hospital. We don't have enough time (or staff) to do it that way."

The nurse who wants to become a leader must be willing to try new methods, to think new thoughts, to accept new ideas — to change. Change is not easy, for it requires that we exert ourselves mentally and physically. Changes makes us uncomfortable. But only when we become uncomfortable, dissatisfied with ourselves and our practice in nursing, will we make any progress. We find that we do not know everything and that we must learn more. So we have completed a circle and find that now we must start all over again, but this is the process of leadership.

STUDY QUESTIONS

1. Discuss the Decalogue of Leadership in more detail. Look for examples in literature and in your own experience which illustrate how the behavior suggested in each commandment helped a person provide better leadership. Compare the decalogue with the beatitudes given in the beginning of the book.
2. Observe situations illustrating directive leadership and creative leadership. If you do not agree with the type of leadership used in each situation, give your reasons.
3. Compare nursing leadership techniques with administrative and supervisory activities.
4. What personal qualities and characteristics do you consider most important in a leader? Why?
5. How can you give each of your coworkers a "psychological pay-

check?" Find out from several categories of workers what they feel would help them most to do a better job. What do they complain about most?

6. Give specific suggestions of techniques which may be used to stimulate cooperation among staff people, between two departments.

7. How are administration, supervision, and leadership similar? How do they differ?

8. Discuss how the functions of management compare with the administrative activities. How can these be implemented in the leadership given by the professional nurse?

PART TWO BIBLIOGRAPHY

Books

Bennett, A. C.: *Methods Improvement in Hospitals.* J. B. Lippincott Company, Philadelphia, 1964.
Brown, Milon: *Effective Supervision.* The Macmillan Company, New York, 1960.
Close, Guy C.: *Work Improvement.* John Wiley and Sons, Inc., New York, 1960.
Cooper, Joseph D.: *How to Get More Done in Less Time.* Doubleday and Company, Garden City, N.Y., 1962.
Dennis, Lorraine Bradt: *Psychology of Human Behavior for Nurses.* W. B. Saunders Company, Philadelphia, 1962.
Dooher, M. Joseph, Editor, and Marquis, Vivienne, Associate Editor: *Effective Communication on the Job.* American Management Association. New York, 1956.
Drucker, Peter F.: *The Effective Executive.* Harper and Row Publishers, Inc., New York, 1967.
Engstrom, Ted W., and MacKenzie, Alex: *Managing Your Time.* Zondervan Publishing House, Grand Rapids, Michigan, 1967.
Flesch, Rudolf: *The Art of Plain Talk.* Harper and Row Publishers, Inc., New York, 1946.
Gardiner, Glenn, et al.: *Managerial Skills for Supervisors.* Elliot Service Company, Mount Vernon, N.Y., 1960.
Heyel, Carl: *The Supervisor's Basic Management Guide.* McGraw-Hill Book Company, New York, 1965.
Jucius, Michael J., and Schlender, Wm. E.: *Elements of Managerial Action.* Richard D. Irwin, Inc., Homewood, Ill., 1965.
Karlins, Marvin, and Abelson, Herbert I.: *Persuasion.* Springer Publishing Company, Inc., New York, 1970.
Kron, Thora: *Communication in Nursing.* W. B. Saunders Company, Philadelphia, 1967.
Lesnik, Milton J., and Anderson, Bernice E.: *Nursing Practice and the Law.* J. B. Lippincott Company, Philadelphia, 1962.
Maslow, A. H.: *Motivation and Personality.* Harper and Row Publishers, Inc., New York, 1954.
Maslow, A. H.: *Toward a Psychology of Being.* 2nd ed. Van Nostrand-Reinhold Books, New York, 1968.
Mason, Joseph G.: *How to Build Your Management Skills.* McGraw-Hill Book Company, New York, 1965.
Osborn, Alex F.: *Applied Imagination.* Charles Scribner's Sons, New York, 1957.
Pieper, Frank: *Modular Management and Human Leadership.* Methods Press, Minneapolis, 1958.
Tead, Ordway: *The Art of Leadership.* McGraw-Hill Book Company, Inc., New York, 1935.
Uris, Auren: *Techniques of Leadership.* McGraw-Hill Book Company, Inc., New York, 1953.

Pamphlets and Journals

About Being a Leader. Monthly Letter of the Royal Bank of Canada, Montreal, Oct. 3, 1957.

Are We Nursing the Patient—or the Paper Work? RN, *27*:12:54, Dec., 1954.

Campbell, Emily B.: *The Process of Change.* Am. J. Nursing, *67*:5:991, May, 1967.

Christman, Luther B.: *Nursing Leadership—Style and Substance.* Am. J. Nursing, *67*:10:2091, Oct., 1967.

Corona, Dorothy F.: *Sedatives and Stimulants to Creativity.* Nurs. Outlook, *12*:7:24, July, 1964.

Davis, Anne J.: *The Skills of Communication.* Am. J. Nursing, *63*:1:66, Jan., 1963.

DeStefano, Grace M.: *Management Program Increases Nursing Service Effectiveness.* Hospital Progress, Dec., 1968, pg. 54.

Dunn, Helen: *Facing Realities in Nursing Administration Today.* Am. J. Nursing, *68*:5:1013, May, 1968.

Egolf, Marion G.: *Unit Management Program Provides More Effective Use of Personnel.* Hospitals, *43*:14:77, July 16, 1969.

Francis, Gloria M.: *How Do I Feel About Myself?* Am. J. Nursing, *67*:6:1244, June, 1967.

Gilbreth, Lillian: *The Basic Questions of Management.* Hospital Progress, *42*:1:55, Jan., 1961.

Ginsberg, Frances: *How to Motivate People to Accept Change.* Modern Hospital, *111*:5:114, Nov., 1968.

Hannan, C. Phillip: *Planning and Implementing a Workable Unit Management System.* Hospital Progress, May, 1969, pg. 120.

Hershey, Nathan: *A Nurse's Liability for Negligence in Supervision.* Am. J. Nursing, *62*:5:115, May, 1962.

How to Study Nursing Activities in a Patient Unit. U.S. Dept. of Health, Education, and Welfare, Publication No. 370, Rev. 1964.

In Pursuit of Efficiency. The Royal Bank of Canada Monthly Letter, *50*:7:1, July, 1969.

In Pursuit of Quality—Hospital Nursing Services. National League for Nursing, Dep't of Hospital Nursing, 1964.

Jimm, Louise R., and Fine, Jerry Hargadine: *A Shared Experience in Leadership.* Nurs. Outlook, *15*:10:36, Oct., 1967.

Lehman, Katherine B.: *Supervision—Variations on a Theme.* Am. J. Nursing, *67*:6:1204, June, 1967.

Margarella, Sister Mary: *Communication: The Catalyst.* Hospital Progress, *41*:5:106, May, 1960.

Mercadante, Lucille: *Utilization—A Vehicle for the Effective Delivery of Patient Care Services.* Minnesota Nursing Accent, Minnesota Nurses' Ass'n, *42*:1:5, Jan., 1970.

Merton, Robert K.: *The Social Nature of Leadership.* Am. J. Nursing, *69*:12:2614, Dec., 1969.

Moore, Larry F.: *Problem Recognition in Nursing Service Administration.* Nursing Forum, *8*:1:94, 1969.

O'Donovan, Thomas R.: *Effective Supervision Requires Leadership.* Hospital Progress, Feb., 1965, page 65.

On Being a Manager. The Royal Bank of Canada Monthly Letter, *51*:2:1, Feb., 1970.

Oshin, Edith S.: *How to Argue Without Losing Your Head.* RN, *25*:10:81, Oct., 1962.

Perkins, Ralph: *The Do's and Don'ts of Delegation.* Hospitals, *36*:17:40, Sept., 1962.

Pollock, Ted: *Put Your Ideas Across Effectively.* Hospital Management, *99*:5:68, May, 1965.

Quest for Quality: A Self-Evaluation Guide to Patient Care. National League for Nursing, Dep't of Hospital Nursing, 1966.

Ramphal, Marjorie: *Clinical Nursing Supervision.* Am. J. Nursing. *68*:9:1900, Sept., 1968.

Robinette, Taskerk: *What Is Health Planning?* Nurs. Outlook, *18*:1:33, Jan., 1970.

Rutherford, Ruby: *What Bothers Staff Nurses?* Am. J. Nursing, *67*:2:315, Feb., 1967.

Sells, Annabell C.: *The First Line Supervisors and Human Relations.* Canadian Nurse, *61*:4:283, April, 1965.

Siggins, Clara M.: *A Professor of English Looks at Communication Skills.* Nurs. Outlook, *9*:11:66, Nov., 1961.

Skarupa, Jack A.: *Management by Objectives—A Systematic Way to Manage Change.* Hospitals, *43*:18:49, Sept. 16, 1969.

Skipper, James K., et al.: *Some Barriers to Communication.* Nursing Forum, *2*:1:14, July, 1963.

Smith, Carol Anne: *Job Satisfaction in Hospital Nursing.* Canadian Nurse, *59*:2:147, Feb., 1963.

Smith, James L.: *The Computer—Its Impact on the Physician, the Nurse, and the Administration.* Hospitals, *43*:18:63, Sept. 16, 1969.

Villeneuve, Jacques P.: *Development of Human Resources.* Canadian Nurse, *61*:2:94, Feb., 1965.

Walker, Virginia, and Hawkins, James L.: *Management: A Factor in Clinical Nursing.* Nurs. Outlook, *13*:2:57, Feb., 1965.

Wolfe, Ilse: *What's in a Word?* Nurs. Outlook, *12*:12:36, Dec., 1964.

Young, Lucie S. *Nursing's Challenge.* Nurs. Outlook. *17*:5:62, May, 1969.

PART THREE

Putting Your Leadership Skills to Work

To look is one thing.
To see what you look at is another.
To understand what you see is a third.
To learn from what you understand is something else . . .
But to act on what you learn is all that really matters!

From the letterhead of Benjamin Pucket,
former president of Allied Stores Corporation

Chapter 7

How to Plan for Patient Care

Nurses must become skillful in the use of the nursing process, i.e., assessment, planning, implementing, and evaluating the care needed by and given to their patients. Planning is based upon assessment — assessment of patient needs, of the staff and their capabilities, and of the facilities available for use in providing care of the patient.

Planning must come before action. If you want to give effective care to your patients, you must give much thought to the planning of that care. As indicated previously, planning is determining a course of action. Neglect in planning is one of the main reasons for confusion and disorganization in ward activities and for poor patient care. As the care of patients becomes more complex, planning becomes more important.

Planning involves making decisions which presuppose the availability of various actions from which to choose. The decisions you make will be influenced by your personal philosophy about your responsibility for the care of your patients and for helping other staff members contribute to that care.

ESSENTIAL PARTS OF A PATIENT CARE PLAN

Today nursing care is defined as the action that the nurse takes in fulfilling her primary function. Yet, as discussed previously, the nurse also gives care which is prescribed by the doctor or dictated by hospital policy; therefore, to differentiate between this delegated care and nursing care, the term *patient care* is used here to describe *all* care for which the nurse is responsible. Patient care includes three aspects: general care which may be prescribed by the doctor or set by hospital policy, medical care which is prescribed by the doctor but delegated to others, and nursing care which the nurse, functioning as an independent practitioner, determines is necessary to help her patient.

General Patient Care. Food and fluid requirements, amount of physical activity, and personal hygiene, safety, and comfort measures may be determined by the patient's illness and the doctor's plan of therapy; however, the time that meals are served or the bath given is often a matter of hospital policy. These aspects of patient care are usually recorded under the heading of general care or general nursing measures.

Delegated Medical Care. The physician's primary responsibility is diagnosis and treatment of illness; however, he delegates specific techniques which are based upon his plan for diagnosis and aim of medical therapy. Those aspects of patient care for which the nurse is not responsible, except to see that they are done, e.g., laboratory tests or physiotherapy, may be listed separately under other headings. The general care and delegated medical care sections of the patient's care plan are commonly found on the treatment and medication part of the Kardex.

Nursing Care or Nursing Intervention. Each patient responds in a different way to illness and its treatment, to his social environment and economic state. He may not even show the same response consistently day after day. He has his own peculiar likes, dislikes, worries, and fears.

Although the nurse works within the dictates of the plan of medical care and of established hospital policy, she must identify the needs and nursing problems of her patient and determine how to meet them. In other words, she makes a nursing diagnosis and prescribes the nursing care needed to solve each nursing problem. These suggestions may be called nursing orders and should be written on the patient's nursing care plan section of the Kardex.

Nursing care may be related to some part of the delegated medical care, e.g., determining what is causing a patient's discomfort and what should be done to make him more comfortable. Nursing care is also needed to adapt a general hospital routine to fit the needs of the individual patient, e.g., selecting the best time and method to make him comfortable for sleep. Nursing care is that help given to the patient to assist him through his illness by minimizing as much as possible the source of his tensions, providing solace, sympathy, and support when needed, and helping him to understand his condition and his treatment and to participate in his care as much as he is able in order to achieve the ultimate aim of the medical and nursing care.

In order to give nursing care every person on the nursing staff must know as much as possible about the patient. In some cases, the nurse will need to use all her knowledge and skill to determine what the patient wants or needs and how to take care of him. In other cases, planning and giving nursing care may be quite simple. Always the entire staff work together in giving this care.

PURPOSES OF THE NURSING CARE PLAN

The nursing care plan shows what the nursing staff is to accomplish for the patient and how to help the patient, including his family, reach these goals by himself. It also directs the staff as to how they may go about achieving these hoped for results most effectively.

To Indicate the Aim of Nursing Care. The aim of nursing care should include the broad or long-term goal and one or more specific or short-term objectives which will help achieve the ultimate result. These are based upon the nurse's assessment of the patient and her nursing diagnosis of his needs. The aim must also take cognizance of the aim of medical therapy.

The patient's diagnosis, religion, marital status, age and so forth are usually written somewhere on the record of the patient's care plan. While this information is not directly a part of the plan, it is important because it provides background material that will help the staff understand the patient better.

To Provide a Guide to Patient-centered Care. One of the main reasons for making a nursing care plan is to provide a guide for patient-centered, rather than job-centered, care. The plan provides information about the problems and needs of the patient and suggestions about how to meet them. The patient is always considered first. His disease is important only to the extent that it affects the physical and emotional aspects of his nursing care.

To Provide a Means of Communication. Another reason for the written care plan is to provide a means of communication to all personnel. In this way, everyone caring for the patient will receive the benefit of the plan and will be better able to carry on a program of continuous individualized care. Continuity of care is important to the patient. The written nursing care plan is the only sure way that the information is available to the staff. The written plan is valuable to each worker, especially the professional nurse, as an introduction to the patient and the care given by preceding workers.

To Provide a Guide for Supervision. Since the plan gives information about what nursing care is needed and how it is to be given, it provides the professional nurse with a guide for her supervision of her staff. By using the plan she can make certain that each patient receives the nursing care that is important to him.

To Provide a Basis for Evaluating Nursing Care. Because the nursing profession does not yet agree on a specific definition of nursing care, nurses tend to evaluate their care on the basis of proficiency in techniques alone. Yet the nurse should evaluate both the quality and quantity of *nursing* care provided by her coworkers. A well-made nursing care plan defines the care for the individual patient or at least a part of it. By referring to this plan, she can begin her evaluation by asking herself, "How well did we meet the needs of this patient as suggested in the nursing care plan?"

THE NURSING PROCESS AND PROBLEM-SOLVING

We have already discussed the steps used in the nursing process and problem-solving. The nursing process is applying problem-solving techniques in the planning of nursing care. We start with the patient and obtain as much information as possible about him and his health needs and problems. This assessment leads to identification of the patient's problems, i.e., the making of a nursing diagnosis. The next step is looking for the various ways that can be used to help this patient, followed by the selection of specific methods to solve each problem. We then have a nursing care plan; however, the suggested care must be used according to the directions if the patient is to receive any benefit. His response to this care must be evaluated to determine whether the best nursing action was selected or whether we should continue to search for another way of helping the patient solve his problems.

GUIDES TO PLANNING NURSING INTERVENTION OR NURSING CARE

While it is not the aim of this book to give detailed instruction about the various guides and techniques which may be used to determine solutions to nursing or patient problems, a brief review could prove helpful at this time.

Needs. One of the most valuable guides is based upon the needs of the individual. Maslow* grouped these into five categories arranged in the order of their importance to the individual in carrying out life processes. These categories are summarized in Figure 5.

---

*Maslow, A. H.: *Motivation and Personality.* Harper and Row Publishers, Inc., New York, 1954.

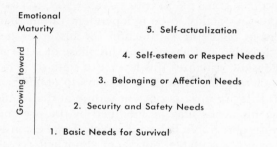

Figure 5. Maslow's hierarchy of needs.

PHYSIOLOGICAL OR SURVIVAL NEEDS. These include oxygen, food, fluids, elimination of body wastes, activity and rest, and sexual satisfaction, with oxygen being the most important. Activity and rest usually refer to physical motion, but perhaps mental activity and rest should also be considered since such activity occurs continuously during life and affects the basic drives. The need for physical comfort, while not absolutely necessary for survival, directly affects the other needs found on this level. It might be placed here or in the next group of needs.

SECURITY OR SAFETY NEEDS. This group of needs has been summarized as the need for economic or job security, for emotional security, spiritual security, and physical safety including comfort. The patient wants to know with some degree of reliability and consistency what is going to happen to him and how he will be affected.

AFFECTION OR BELONGING NEEDS. These needs include those for love, for kindness and consideration from others, for feeling a part of a family or group. In functioning on this level the individual begins to give to others as well as receive from them.

ESTEEM OR RECOGNITION NEEDS. This level is related to the one preceding. Status and reputation within the group become important. However, satisfaction on this level depends on the degree of emotional maturity achieved, i.e., the stage of *becoming.* In the beginning the individual gets his satisfaction from the approval and respect shown to him by other people. Later his satisfaction is influenced by the degree of self-respect he has acquired based upon how he views himself as a person and how he values his capabilities. As he achieves emotional maturity his satisfaction of these needs stems from his sense of mastery and competency in daily life and work. He becomes interested in people and respects them as individuals.

SELF-DETERMINING OR SELF-ACTUALIZATION NEEDS. These include the person's ability to be independent rather than dependent upon others in obtaining satisfaction for his other needs. He becomes self-directive and moves into the phase of self-fulfillment and creativity. Maslow visualizes this level as a state of *being* oneself.

A person may use a number of ways to obtain satisfaction for those needs that are most important to him at the moment. His way of satisfying his needs may be modified by the presence of disease and will cause observable behavior which may be considered either acceptable or not acceptable, normal or abnormal, according to standards set up by society. For example, he may try to get attention by loud talking, by rowdy behavior, or by constantly demanding services from those around him. He may substitute one need that he is able to satisfy for another which he is unable to satisfy; e.g., the compulsive eater may be one who is unable to obtain as much love or affection as he desires. It is also possible either to overemphasize a need or to deny it completely, e.g., to constantly require approval from other people or to ignore completely the opinion of others around him.

As nurses we recognize that during times of stress, such as illness, an individual tends to regress, i.e., operate on a level closer to the base of the hierarchy than to the self-actualizing level. He will be relatively unconcerned with what people think of him when he is in pain; or when he is afraid, he will seek security from the nursing staff by putting on his call light frequently.

21 Nursing Problems. Another valuable guide to the planning of nursing care is the 21 Nursing Problems* listed below. The nurse may use these as nursing problems to be solved or as aims of nursing care to be achieved through identification of more specific nursing or patient problems.

1. To maintain good hygiene and physical comfort.
2. To promote optimal activity: exercise, rest, and sleep.
3. To promote safety through prevention of accident, injury, or other trauma and through the prevention of the spread of infection.
4. To maintain good body mechanics and prevent and correct deformities.
5. To facilitate the maintenance of a supply of oxygen to all body cells.
6. To facilitate the maintenance of nutrition to all body cells.
7. To facilitate the maintenance of elimination.
8. To facilitate the maintenance of fluid and electrolyte balance.
9. To recognize the physiological responses of the body to disease conditions—pathological, physiological, and compensatory.
10. To facilitate the maintenance of regulatory mechanisms and functions.

---

*Abdellah, Faye G., Beland, Irene L., Martin, Almeda, and Matheney, Ruth V.: *Patient-centered Approaches to Nursing.* © Copyright, The Macmillan Co., 1960.

11. To facilitate the maintenance of sensory function.

12. To identify and accept positive and negative expressions, feelings, and reactions.

13. To identify and accept the interrelatedness of emotions and organic illness.

14. To facilitate the maintenance of effective verbal and nonverbal communication.

15. To promote the development of productive interpersonal relationships.

16. To facilitate progress toward achievement of personal spiritual goals.

17. To create and/or maintain a therapeutic environment.

18. To facilitate awareness of self as an individual with varying physical, emotional, and developmental needs.

19. To accept the optimum possible goals in the light of limitations, physical and emotional.

20. To use community resources as an aid in resolving problems arising from illness.

21. To understand the role of social problems as influencing factors in the cause of illness.

The needs described in the previous paragraphs are enlarged upon in this list of nursing problems. The aims and plan of medical therapy will, of course, influence the methods that the nurse decides to use in meeting these needs or solving the problems.

Health Strengths and Limitations. Bonney and Rothberg* use this method of assessment in order to identify the various problems of the patient. In their method the nurse lists the strengths or assets of the patient, that which he is able and willing to do for himself or what he understands. Then she lists the weaknesses or limitations of the patient, that which he is unable or unwilling to do for himself or what he does not accept or understand. The patient needs help in overcoming these limitations. When planning his care, the nurse will try to use some of his strengths to help him overcome his weaknesses.

HOW TO PLAN INDIVIDUALIZED NURSING CARE

Perhaps a word should be said first about what should and should not be included in the plan. In general, the plan should include:

1. Problems concerning the giving of delegated medical care.
2. Problems which affect the method of doing any nursing technique or the carrying out of any responsibility delegated by the doctor.

---

*Bonney, Virginia and Rothberg, June: *Nursing Diagnosis and Therapy.* National League for Nursing, 1963.

3. Problems concerning information to be given to the patient or to his relatives.
4. Problems which affect the interpersonal relationships between patient and worker.
5. Problems concerning the patient's response to his environment, his illness, and his inability to care for himself.
6. Suggestions for possible solutions to the problems. These approaches must be developed for the individual patient.

In general the plan should not include:

1. Confidential information about the patient.
2. Suggestions for approaches which are repetitions of hospital routines or of doctor's orders.

Identifying Needs, Patient Problems, and Nursing Problems. Needs and problems are not identical, although one grows out of, or is related to, the other. Needs are concerned with the processes necessary for life and with the person's response to his environment. A problem arises when a conflict occurs between one or more of these needs, either because of the effect of disease on the body or because the patient uses an unacceptable way to fulfill a need. For example, the body needs water if it is to carry on its life processes. What happens if the patient is nauseated and refuses all food and fluids; if he is willing to drink but is unable to do so because of mouth surgery; or if he is limited in his fluid intake but insists on drinking too much? In each case, the need and the problem involve the fluid intake of the patient; however, in each situation, the cause of the problem is different. Therefore, the solution must be specific for the cause and thus individualized for the patient.

Perhaps an illustration will help. We had a patient who had polyneuritis, causing the loss of motion in both his arms. This physical symptom may be called behavior in that it is the body's response to a disease process.

Planning the nursing care for this patient may be approached either by using the hierarchy of needs approach or by using the 21 Nursing Problems. When using the needs approach, the nurse may ask the question, "How does this physical symptom (this behavior) affect the patient's need for food, fluids, and so forth (or for job security)? In using the nursing problem approach, she may ask, "How may I maintain good hygiene and physical comfort and promote optimal activity for this patient?"

To illustrate the planning of care using the needs approach, how does this physical symptom affect each of the following needs?

1. The patient's need for food.

He must have food, but his ability to feed himself has been lost; therefore, the nurse must do for the patient what he is unable to do for himself. To individualize this care the nurse should determine his likes and dislikes for food and how he wants to be fed.

2. The patient's need for fluids.

   He must have fluids, but he cannot reach for the glass himself. Furthermore, he is unable to use the call light when he feels thirsty. Perhaps the nurse is creative enough to rig up some way that the patient can use a bell with either his head or his feet; otherwise, she may decide to check him at stated intervals.

3. The patient's need for elimination of body waste.

   Elimination of wastes takes place through the skin, lungs, bladder, and intestinal tract. The patient's self-esteem may also be a factor, for he may be so embarrassed about asking a nurse to place the urinal or bedpan that he will not ask for it until absolutely necessary. Part of the nurse's responsibility is prevention of complications, so she must take steps to prevent constipation or retention of urine which might predispose to urinary tract infection or other difficulties.

4. The patient's need for oxygen.

   His inability to use his arms affects his moving about in bed, which in turn may lead to shallow respirations and accumulation of secretions in the lungs. Furthermore, bed rest with pressure on body prominences may cut off blood supply, i.e., oxygen and nutrition, to tissue cells, so the nurse must plan how to ensure an adequate supply of nutrition and oxygen reaching all parts of the body, thereby preventing decubiti.

Needs or Problems	Approach	Evaluation
3/15 Unable to feed self	Feed patient. Wife comes for eve. meal. Milk for dinner and supper. Feed all of one food before starting another.	3/16 Eating well.
3/15 Unable to call nurses	Check q½h. Offer fluids. Plan for at least 1500 cc intake between 7 A.M. and 7 P.M.	3/17 Intake low
3/15 Hesitates to ask for urinal or bedpan	Offer urinal and bedpan. Usually has B.M. before breakfast. Don't leave on pan for long time. Give prune je. daily.	3/18 Urinary output good. No B.M. for 3 days. Laxative given. Good results.
3/15 Prevent breakdown of tissue	Turn, cough, and breathe deeply when giving special care as per schedule.	3/19 Skin in good condition
3/15 States: "I am no good to anyone."	Allow him to decide about his care. Ask his opinion. Stress any improvement.	3/18 Continues to be depressed

5. The patient's need to feel worthwhile and to have respect for himself.

The loss of physical ability or a disturbance in health may cause a person to lose some of his self-esteem because he may believe that others will think less of him. The nursing problem is to select ways that will bolster the patient's self-esteem.

This patient had many personal and nursing problems, but these are the main ones that could be listed on the nursing care plan. From these suggestions you can readily see how the approach can be made using the 21 Nursing Problems as a guide to arrive at basically the same nursing care plan shown in the chart on page 103.

When care is given according to an established routine or procedure, there is no need to repeat the schedule on the care plan. It may be necessary to indicate where the information may be found.

To identify patient and nursing problems by assessment of strengths and limitations, the nurse may proceed in this way.

Strengths	*Limitations*
1. Anxious to get well. Tries to help as much as possible. 2. Health was good before this. 3. Wife is accepting added responsibility very well.	1. Unable to move arms. 2. Will not ask for personal care unless absolutely necessary. 3. Depressed. Thinks he is not of any use any more.

Some of the problem areas are the same, but the information included in the strengths gives an additional source of help to the nurse as she plans the care of this patient.

There are no set forms for a nursing care plan although a number of forms are available from commercial printing companies. The nurse should realize that evaluation of nursing measures is a necessary part of the nursing process and these notations can be made on the nursing care plan to help in revising the plan of care.

The question is sometimes asked whether the doctor must be informed of nursing problems and must agree to the proposed solutions. The aims of the health team, of which both doctor and nurse are members, are to aid in the recovery of the patient and to return him to his home and community where he may function to the limit of his ability. As members of this health team the doctor and nurse cannot afford to function as separate entities. Any problem affecting the patient is the concern of both, and the aim of nursing care cannot be separated from the aim of medical treatment. There must always be communication between doctor and nurse.

Whether the doctor must approve the solutions to the patient's problems as proposed by the nursing staff will depend upon two factors. First, it will depend on whether the approach is merely a modification of an accepted hospital policy or nursing procedure or whether it involves some aspect of the medical treatment instituted by the doctor. Secondly, it will depend on the amount of rapport existing between the doctor and nurse and the confidence he has in her use of good judgment.

Suppose the problem involves helping the patient to increase his fluid intake. Perhaps the first approach would be to find out what fluids this patient particularly likes and, therefore, would drink more readily. The problem of adequate fluid intake certainly should be called to the attention of the doctor; however, the nurse's approach at this point does not need his approval. After the nurse finds out what the patient likes, the solution to the problem may be changed to the provision of those fluids which he prefers. Since this is probably accepted hospital procedure, it does not need to be approved by the doctor, although the nurse will undoubtedly want to keep him informed. On the other hand, if the nurse finds out that the patient likes some fluids contraindicated by the medical treatment, the doctor must decide whether to change his treatment; therefore, the proposed solution is brought to the doctor's attention and must receive his approval before it can be used.

Determining the Objectives of Nursing Care. The aim of nursing care is found in the needs and problems of the patient and may be related either to his inability, because of some problem, to satisfy one or more of his basic needs or to the aim of medical treatment instituted by the doctor. The statement of the objective must be specific to the patient and cannot be merely a repetition of a general aim of care for every patient. For example, the aims, "keep the patient comfortable" and "help the patient learn to care for himself" or "to recover without complications," are common to every patient in the hospital. The objective must be related to what the nursing staff hope to accomplish as they care for each particular person. "Keep the patient comfortable" would be an acceptable objective of nursing care only if he is suffering from intractable pain and if the main aim of medical therapy is the alleviation of that pain.

There is no need to list an objective of care for every problem. Rather the objective should be worded in such a way that the most important problem or problems are indicated. For example, "help the patient adjust to his loss of vision" and "help the patient to accept his colostomy and learn how to care for it" indicate the areas where major problems exist for these patients and what the staff hope to accomplish through their approach to each problem.

Short-term or more specific aims of care should also be suggested. These are selected as steps toward reaching the broad or long-range goal. For example, for the patient who has lost his sight, "help the patient learn to feed himself" or "help him to learn to move around his room" are stepping stones to the final goal of adjustment to his blindness.

Planning patient-centered care is not easy but, with practice, you and your coworkers will become better able to consider each patient as an individual, to define his problems and to determine the best way to meet those problems. The quality of nursing care resulting from this kind of planning is a constant source of satisfaction to you and your coworkers, as well as to your patients. In addition, it provides a challenge to improve your knowledge and understanding as you care for each new patient.

HOW TO BEGIN THE NURSING CARE PLAN

Begin When the Patient Is Admitted. The nursing care plan should be started when the patient enters the hospital. Although the nurse may delegate the admission techniques and the processing of the first orders to someone else, she must visit the patient and make her own observations.

Some hospitals are including in the admission routine the use of a structured interview or a nursing admission interview form which becomes part of the patient's record. When the nurse visits the patient during the admission period, she uses this interview method to get enough information in order to start planning individual care. The purpose of this interview is to get to know the patient. The form may list various questions such as the following:

1. Have you been in a hospital before? When? Why?
2. What makes you feel comfortable when you are sick?
3. Are you on any special medication?
4. Do you have any allergies?
5. Do you have any special likes or dislikes about food?
6. Do you have any difficulty sleeping?
7. Do you have any difficulty in bowel elimination? In elimination of urine?
8. Do you want any restriction on visitors?

These questions should suggest others that could be asked. The questions should be planned according to the age and condition of the patient; e.g., the nurse could ask the parents of a small child about special words he uses to express his wants, or about the schedule of activities he is used to at home.

As the nurse talks with the patient, she should observe his appearance, facial expression, speech, and behavior. When she has completed the interview and received reports from anyone else who has been with the patient, she is ready to begin the nursing care plan for the patient.

How to Start the Nursing Care Plan.   This initial plan is based on the treatment instituted by the doctor and upon any information obtained by you or any other person who helped with the admission of the patient. Perhaps you observe that the patient is hard of hearing or a relative tells you that the patient has been incontinent at home. Write the problem or problems on the nursing care plan along with your suggestions for solving them. If the patient has a hearing aid or can read lips, note it on the plan. If you foresee the possibility of bedsores because of the incontinence, plan now to prevent them. If the doctor ordered the insertion of an indwelling catheter, the incontinence is no longer a nursing problem. Instead, you foresee the possibility of other problems occurring, such as keeping the catheter working properly or minimizing urethral irritation. Perhaps when you give the first dose of medicine, the patient informs you that he cannot swallow pills; here is another problem. So you record the appropriate approach on the care plan or on the medication card, indicating that the tablets must be crushed. You have made a good start already toward individualizing the care of this patient. During these initial observations, you should look for evidence of fear or apprehension in the patient toward his hospitalization, evidence of loss of sight, or any language difficulties. Record what the patient states to be his likes and dislikes, or what he is allergic to. With practice you will find many other areas of information that can easily be included within this period of admitting the patient and starting his treatment. This initial plan may also include the teaching needs of the patient. For example, he should be taught about the tests and examinations ordered for him or about the turning and breathing exercises he must do after surgery.

The listing of any definite problems you see at this time is just as important as the listing of the medications and treatments ordered by the doctor if you are to provide total care of this patient. Later, after your staff has become acquainted with the patient, you will further assess his condition and problems.

HOW TO KEEP NURSING CARE PLANS UP TO DATE

When we are working with people, we cannot expect a situation to remain unchanged. Assessment of needs must be a continuous process. Consequently the nursing care plan will change as the patient's needs or nursing problems change.

Every professional nurse is responsible for initiating the nursing care plan and for keeping it up to date. This includes the head nurse and every staff nurse. Any nursing care plan, if it is to be effective, must contain information concerning the care the patient needs at the present time. This present care will also include the foreseeing of future problems and trying to prevent them. Anything that is not related to the patient's present care should be removed from the care plan. Some problems will be solved and new ones will appear because the patient's condition is always changing. Even the long-term patient will present new problems, since, even though they may be barely discernible, physical and emotional changes occur in response to confinement and disability.

Daily nursing conferences, keeping the care plans up to date and using them constantly are the prerequisites for effective nursing care. Current information is necessary if the plan of care is to be of any value to you or to your staff and especially to the patient. You must find the times when it is most convenient for you to bring the information up to date.

During Rounds to Visit Your Patients.   As you visit each of your patients, you may receive information, either from what you see or from what the patient tells you, indicating that a change in his plan of care is necessary. If the change is slight, you can make the adjustment immediately. Perhaps a patient requests that his leg be placed in a certain position when he is sitting in a chair. If that position is not contraindicated, note the patient's request on his care plan immediately. If for any reason his request cannot be granted, you must take care of the problem at once by giving him sufficient information for him to understand why it is impossible to do as he has requested. In addition you must determine what different approach will be acceptable and also solve his problem.

When the Kardex and Patient's Chart Are Checked.   The Kardex and each patient's chart are checked at regular intervals to insure that no information is omitted. Usually this is part of the administrative responsibility of the head nurse; however, she may at this time find areas in the care plan which should be changed or have suggestions concerning additional care for the patient. This is especially true if the doctor has changed his plan of treatment. If part of your responsibility involves taking care of the doctor's orders for your patients, remember that it is just as important to check the special problems of the patient as it is to check the plan for his treatments.

When a Report Is Given.   One of the most common times for bringing the care plan up to date is at the time of a report. Usually when one shift reports to the next is the time when the professional nurse may offer her suggestions concerning the nursing care she feels the patient needs. She may also report her observations concerning the effectiveness of the various approaches being used. In this way, the private duty nurse is made to feel that she contributes to the nursing care plan even though she may not actually work with it.

During any report, the entire plan should be noted, not just that part concerned with the doctor's orders. For example, if, during a report about a patient, you note that the indwelling catheter about which there was a problem has been taken out, the notations must be removed from both places in the patient care plan. On the other hand, if you foresee that the removal of the catheter may cause new problems, perhaps that of incontinence or of insuring that the patient is voiding in adequate amounts, this new problem should be noted on the plan at this time, as well as your suggested approach. This new information is then included in your reports to your co-workers and to your head nurse.

At the Nursing Conference.   Although you may make changes in the plan of care whenever you find it necessary, nothing can take the place of the conference for complete evaluation and planning by the entire group. This is the time for a complete review of the patient's care to insure that all parts of the plan are usable and that nothing has been omitted.

QUESTIONS ASKED ABOUT NURSING CARE PLANS

How can I convince the nursing personnel of the usefulness and importance of the care plans? The nursing care plan can be just as useful as you want it to be. The personnel will more readily see its value if the plan is carefully thought out and made individual for the patient. Then the plan will help them in their work. Refer to the plan whenever you talk about the patient. Use it in planning your work and when you help your staff to plan their work. Refer to it again to determine if their work has been done properly. When the members of your team see you using the plans continuously, they will use them too.

How can you make out the nursing care plan when you don't have time to talk to the patient? It is impossible to plan the nursing care for the individual unless you are acquainted with him. I believe there are two aspects of this problem that you should consider. First, are you sure that you can't find time to talk *with* the patient? I am sure that you must come to his bedside several times during the day; otherwise, you are not assuming your responsibilities as a professional nurse. The problem then becomes one of making the best use of these few minutes, to talk *with*, not *to*, your patient, getting him to talk about himself. You should never allow yourself to become so busy that you do not see or hear the patient as you give him his medicine, put on his hot packs, irrigate his catheter, change his dressings, or make your rounds.

The second aspect of this problem is directly related to one of the reasons for having a nursing care conference. Knowing that you do not have as much time as you would like to become acquainted with the patient, you then must rely upon the eyes and ears of your coworkers. You need to become skillful in questioning them so that they will relate as many details as possible about the patients. As conference leader, you have the great responsibility, first, of collecting all the information the nursing staff may have; and secondly, of determining the importance of their information in relation to the care the patient needs.

How can the nursing care plan be made more individual for each patient? In order to make the plan individual you must know as much as possible about your patient—his disease and how it affects him, his treatment, his likes and dislikes, his home and family, and his worries in order to determine his needs and nursing problems.

Where should the nursing care plans be kept? Since the plan for nursing care is only one part of the patient care plan, it must be kept with the rest of the plan, i.e., in the Kardex. Realizing that the Kardex is used frequently, you will need to discuss the information about the nursing care plan at the same time that you discuss the medical care responsibilities (treatments and medications) delegated to you by the physician.

Should everyone on the nursing staff read the nursing care plan? Absolutely. If each person is to contribute to the total care of the patient, she must know what and how to do it. Certainly the nursing care plan should not be the jealously guarded secret of just a few persons. In fact the patient himself should be made a contributing member in making his plan of care.

STUDY QUESTIONS

1. Select two patients. Using one or more of the suggested guides to the planning of nursing care as described on pages 98 to 104, identify the specific needs and nursing problems for your patients, and suggest possible approaches to the nursing care of your patients. Be sure to consider all their needs in relation to their disease conditions and their symptoms. Then make a nursing care plan for each patient.

2. While you admit a patient, obtain as much information as you can. Start a care plan for this patient.

3. What are the various reasons for having a written nursing care plan?

4. What are the essential parts of a patient care plan? Discuss the ways in which information can be obtained for each part of the plan.

5. List the times and the methods that can be used on your sections to keep the nursing care plans up to date.

6. Select a number of patients and evaluate their care plans. How much individualized care is indicated? What approaches seem good? Why? Which approaches could be improved? How? Is the aim of nursing care consistent with the problems of the patient or with the plan of therapy ordered by the doctor?

Chapter 8

How to Conduct a Nursing Care Planning Conference

PURPOSES OF THE CONFERENCE

The group discussion and nursing care plan tend to eliminate the old functional method of care because all staff members are more aware of the patient as a person and how they can help him. Here you have the opportunity to encourage group dynamics and teamwork. Here also your staff are able to find the answers to their questions concerning the patients, their diseases, and their care. The conferences should be helpful and gratifying to you and to each member of your group. The patient benefits because of the consideration given to him when the group plans care specifically for him.

To Plan the Care of the Individual Patient. The emphasis during the discussion is placed on the patient and the nursing care he needs. Any explanation of his disease is incidental and is given only when necessary to help the inexperienced members of the group understand the patient's symptoms, behavior, or treatment. For example, they should be able to give better care to a patient who has hyperthyroidism when they realize that the patient's desire to have her room kept cool, her extreme restlessness, and large appetite are symptoms of her disease.

When a patient enters the hospital, his doctor is concerned with making a medical diagnosis and developing a plan of therapy. As a nurse, you should also be interested in making a diagnosis, except that your diagnosis is concerned with nursing problems. Your knowledge of the patient's condition and symptoms and how they affect him, combined with your observations and those of your coworkers, must be used to identify these problems. Like the doctor, you are also interested in developing a plan, except that your plan involves the nursing care the patient needs. With the help of your staff, you work out methods of giving this nursing care as well as those aspects of treatment that have been delegated by the physician. Your plan may include the modification of specific nursing procedures, the teaching and encouragement the patient needs, and the way of utilizing the services of the other members of the health team and the community. As the problems of the patient change, his care plan must also be changed.

Continuity in the care of the patient is aided by the discussion during the nursing care conference and by the written nursing care plan, which is a record of the care each patient needs and how it should be given. Therefore, you must stress to each person the importance of using the nursing care plans in her work in order to help the patient to recover as quickly as possible.

The emphasis of this conference must always be on evaluation of patient needs and planning patient care. The discussion must be more than a report about what the person did for each patient; nor is this the time to make assignments or to plan the work for the day.

To Coordinate All Available Services. During the conference, your group becomes aware of the different services offered to the patient by the hospital, by other members of the health team, and by other agencies within the community. As they make use of some of these, they may find additional sources of help for their patients. For example, a patient had some complications following a radical mastectomy; however, she insisted on going home to her family even though she had a profuse drainage. Her husband was afraid that she would injure herself by working too hard, since they were financially unable to hire someone to do the housework and care for the children. The help of the local chapter of the American Cancer Society was enlisted to supply dressings. One of the workers there suggested consulting a group of women from a nearby church who helped in times of sickness by going into the home, doing the heavier housework and looking after the children when necessary. The family was happy with the suggestion, so arrangements were made with the women's group. Thus, by making use of one community agency, the nursing staff discovered another source of help.

To Promote a Spirit of Cooperation. As your staff work together, learning more about their patients, and participating in the planning and giving of their care, the spirit of teamwork is stimulated by the feeling of satisfaction which comes when they are able to do their work well. During the conference, you can also encourage cooperation by constantly stressing the contribution each individual makes toward the care of the patient. No one should be allowed to talk about "my" patients; rather, everyone should be encouraged to speak of "our" patients.

To Increase the Understanding of the Nursing Staff. The ability to work together develops only as each person learns more about what good nursing care is and what her role is in providing that care. Your coworkers will acquire more understanding as you supervise them in the performance of their duties. Supervision is also carried on during the conference. As you observe and listen to the discussion, areas in which the people need more understanding may appear. Some instruction can be given to the entire group during the conference. How to talk with patients, what to say and what not to say, interpretation of hospital policies, the ethics involved in keeping confidential all personal information about the patient—these are only a few topics that may grow out of the discussion of specific problems of a patient.

PLANNING FOR THE CONFERENCE

Some preliminary planning is necessary to keep the conference moving smoothly and to help everyone to benefit by participating in planning the nursing care for their patients.

Planning Individualized Patient Care. The question sometimes arises concerning the value of having a conference if only two people are on duty and each one is caring for different patients. However, there is no set number of people necessary in order to hold a conference. Remember that one of the important responsibilities of the professional nurse is the planning of individualized nursing care. Even one person, such as a night nurse working alone without the assistance of a nurses' aide, should have a part in contributing to the plan of care for any patient. For example, she may leave suggestions concerning specific care that will help the patient rest during the night or that will help other nurses care for the patient. This will give the patient a feeling of security as well as providing for continuity of care.

One head nurse noted that a certain patient was always very restless whenever the regular night nurse was off duty. When she questioned this nurse, the head nurse discovered that the patient liked to be prepared for sleep about twelve o'clock. The regular night nurse always planned her work so that she could spend some time with this patient, rubbing his back, fixing his room as he liked it, and following this with a glassful of warm milk and a cheerful goodnight. The patient would then sleep soundly until his early morning treatment. These were little things, yes, but very important to the patient, who recognized that the other nurses did not know about this part of his care. The patient thought, perhaps unconsciously, that they did not know about the rest of his care; consequently, he became worried and restless. This aspect of care was recorded on the patient's care plan and when everyone followed the same routine, the patient slept well every night; it made no difference which nurse was on duty.

Selecting the Best Time. A time for the conference must be selected with the work of the other personnel in mind since you cannot leave your patients unattended while you are having a conference. Select a time which does not conflict with the work of the other personnel; then stick to it every day. In addition, your co-workers must know where to meet so that each one can arrange her work and be there on time. Soon everyone will accept the conference as part of the day's routine. It is, however, your responsibility to remind them; therefore, post a notice on the station bulletin board, giving the time and the place of the conference along with the name of the patient or patients to be discussed. This information could also be noted on each person's assignment sheet.

The conference does not have to be lengthy. Getting your group together for even 5 or 10 minutes of rapidly moving patient-centered discussion is much better than 20 or 30 minutes of rambling talk. Of course, the more time you have available, the more details you can discuss. However, it is better to start with a short daily conference and increase the time later as you and your coworkers become more adept in using the conference to plan care.

Selecting a Patient. Knowing beforehand which patient will be considered is a very important part of planning for the conference. Ideally, the patient should be chosen the day before the conference, but this may not always be possible. However, this information should be available by the time of the report so that everyone has some time to become acquainted with the patient.

The question of selecting a patient for the conference can be difficult sometimes. Here are some suggestions to consider when making your selection. The patient who has been admitted to the hospital within the last 24 hours needs first consideration. Suppose one has been admitted for diagnosis. Some of the problems that you can readily foresee concern the patient's feelings toward his illness, his fear of the unknown diagnosis, and observations that can be made to help the doctor in making a diagnosis. Perhaps another patient has been admitted to be prepared for surgery during the next few days. Here again some problems may appear to you; for example, the feelings of this patient about the impending surgery and its possible outcome, or the teaching that should be done before surgery. In either case, you need to decide which patient has the more pressing problems. Of course, if you have time, you may wish to consider both patients at the same conference, identifying only the main problem of each patient.

Additional consideration must be given to the fact that a patient's condition is never static. There is always some change and, with that change, some problems may disappear while new ones appear. You must review the progress of each patient. Sometimes even though a patient has recently been discussed, a new and serious problem develops, which was unforeseen at the time of the first conference. You may wish to use one conference to review and revise the nursing care plans for a number of patients. If any of your coworkers report difficulties encountered when giving care to certain patients, the group can discuss and clarify the causes for the difficulties and then develop a satisfactory approach.

Patients who are in the hospital because of a slowly progressive disease, or who have a long convalescence, may be forgotten unless you make it a general rule to periodically evaluate the nursing care needs of these long-term patients. The changes in their conditions may be so indefinite that there seems to be almost none at all. Yet some change always occurs, either emotional or physical, if not both, and with those changes come different problems, which necessitate different approaches.

Frequently, nursing aides will show an interest in a particular patient, not always because of his problems, but because of their interest in his condition or in him as a person. Whenever possible, the group should be allowed to choose the patient or patients they would like to discuss. Their interest will always stimulate more discussion and better planning for individualized care.

Preparation of a Conference Leader. You must make a certain amount of personal preparation for the conference. First of all, you must know as much as possible about the patient and his condition from your own personal observation. You may wish to give a part of his care in order to allow yourself time to talk with him; at least, you will need to visit him. In addition, you may want to spend some time in review of the disease and the reasons for the treatment the physician has ordered. However, you will find before long that, as you increase in experience, your need for this preliminary study will decrease, although you must always review in your own mind what you know about the patient's condition, comparing it with what your staff should know.

The possibility of being unable to answer the questions that their staff may ask causes some nurses to approach the conference with fear and trembling. However, any well-prepared leader should have no qualms in this respect. There is no person in the world who knows everything or is able to answer every question, and the group will not expect that much of their leader.

As part of your own preparation, you should plan the points, preferably in writing, that you want to bring out in the discussion.

Illustration

This is the first conference on Miss Miller, a 77 year old former librarian, whose only complaint is dull back pain, usually in the lumbar area. Her nursing care plan already includes the notations that she likes all juices except grapefruit and apple juice, that she wants to use her own soap for her bath, and that she does not want to be prepared for sleep until after the ten o'clock news. Her doctor has ordered a number of laboratory tests and x-rays.

To help the staff identify other patient and nursing problems, you may suggest that they try to get answers to such questions as:

1. Are there any other likes and dislikes?
2. What questions does she ask?
3. Does she have any physical complaints?
4 Observe her carefully for any forgetfulness, dry skin, poor appetite, or other symptoms.

These questions can be used to start the discussion at the time of the conference. They will also provide a way of helping each person contribute to the nursing care plan and will serve to keep their thoughts centered on this patient and what they can do to help her.

CONDUCTING THE CONFERENCE

Always start the conference on time. Don't wait for the late ones to come, for if you do, they will come later and later each time. When they discover that they are missing something, they will try to be more prompt.

Before starting the discussion, try to make everyone comfortable and at ease. Seating the group in a circle will give the impression of group unity and will encourage each person to participate. Show your interest in each individual and your appreciation for her contribution. Remember that the conference is an informal discussion by the entire group, not a lecture given by the leader.

Starting the Discussion. You may want to begin with a brief review of the patient's condition. Sometimes the temptation is very strong to spend too much time discussing the disease, especially if it is rare or has been difficult to diagnose, or the laboratory tests. Always remember the background of the group and make explanations, if they are absolutely necessary, as brief and simple as possible. Include only that information necessary to explain the patient's needs and problems. If the disease is one with which the people are familiar, you may omit this general information in order to provide more time for considering the problems of the patient.

At another conference, additional information may be given, if the group shows need of it, to increase their understanding of the patient. The conference is not a ward class. It is not concerned primarily with teaching about the treatment and nursing care of a patient who has a certain disease. It is concerned with developing a satisfactory plan to be used as a guide by those who take care of this particular patient.

Now is the time to begin drawing out the information. There are many ways to get this discussion started; for example, you could say, "Let's talk about Miss Miller and what we can do to help her."

From this opening you may get some comments which you, as the conference leader, feel may indicate nursing problems; for example:

1. "She always wants her things put just so on her bedside table."
2. "In the morning she wants to be fixed up first and tells us just what we are to do."
3. "She asks the same questions over and over about what her doctor has ordered for her, then says, 'No one tells me anything.' "

As a professional nurse you can readily see that these comments are related to the needs of the patient for security — to know what is going to happen and to have some control over her environment. She shows evidence of anxiety which you must plan to relieve by giving answers that she can understand. Also, you and your staff can plan her care so that you anticipate her requests.

Responsibilities of the Conference Leader. Leadership is very important during the conference, because the kind of nursing care each patient will receive is based upon the care plan developed by the group. When the leadership is used wisely, they will feel that they are planning the care by themselves. Yet the leader must guide and control her group throughout the entire conference.

Keep the discussion patient-centered. One of your responsibilities is to keep the group thinking about the needs of the specific patient and to keep the discussion "moving forward" toward a solution of his problems. As a rule, you should discourage anyone who tries to bring another patient into the discussion, unless a comparison is being made that will help the group to understand this patient in some specific way. As much as possible, avoid repetition by reminding the group that the information has already been given. Some people find it difficult to speak briefly or to bring out points in a logical order. Sometimes you can help by interrupting with a summarizing statement. If the group begins to digress, bring them back quickly by reminding them of the subject that should be discussed.

Encourage everyone to participate. Throughout the entire

conference, you must provide the opportunity and encouragement for making everyone feel free to participate. At no time should one person, including the leader, do most of the talking. You are to act as moderator and guide, using suggestions and questions to help the group to decide how to give care to a particular patient. When presenting a question for the consideration of the group, give them some time for thought. A moment of silence does not mean that you must answer your own question immediately. Throughout the discussion, you need to recognize the abilities of each person and help each one to improve her ability to express her ideas, to understand the patient and his needs, and to plan his care.

Acknowledge each contribution in such a way that the person is encouraged to participate again. It is easy to give this recognition when her contribution has been correct and valuable; however, a problem arises when her information is incorrect or incomplete. Corrections and additions must be made so that everyone will know what is right, yet care must be taken lest the person become discouraged and not try again. You may meet this situation in a number of ways; for example, if the information is incomplete, you may say:

"Do any of you have anything further to add?" or sometimes simply say, "And?"

"Did you think through the entire question?"

"Let me word the question this way," or "Let's approach the problem from this angle." Then rephrase your original question.

"There is more yet. Can any of you think what it might be?"

"I hadn't thought of that, but it's a good idea. However, I had something else in mind."

If the statement is incorrect, either in part or in whole, you may wish to acknowledge the contribution by saying:

"Most of what you say is correct, but I wonder about . . . ?"

"Do you all agree with that statement?"

"Are you sure that what you are saying is correct?"

"I wonder if you heard the question correctly?"

"I believe that you may have missed the point somewhat. Isn't it true that . . . ?"

"Where did you find your information?"

As a rule, it is wise to avoid asking questions that can be answered by either "Yes" or "No," except when you wish to limit the discussion by a person who talks too much. If you do ask such a question, you may want to follow with the questions "How?" or "Why?" in order to stimulate more discussion.

UTILIZE ALL OPPORTUNITIES FOR TEACHING. While teaching is not the primary purpose of the conference, it can be a valuable outgrowth of the discussion, particularly when it concerns methods for improving the nursing care or areas related to ethics or attitudes. You can do this teaching quite often by means of suggestions or leading questions rather than by dogmatic statements. For example, you could say:

"Do you suppose we could . . . ?"

"Would it be wiser to . . . ?"

"Do you mean that . . . ?"

"Is it possible to . . . ?"

"Your suggestion will work, but . . ."

"How do you think the patient would feel about . . . ?"

"How would you feel if you were the patient?"

Assisting your staff to recognize the problems in nursing care and to develop suitable methods of solving the problems of each patient is your major responsibility. Your group will probably recognize that pain is a problem to a certain patient and may suggest, "Keep the patient comfortable." However, this can be said for many patients. Since your aim is to provide *individualized patient care,* you must help your staff to decide *how* to keep this particular patient comfortable.

Another area in which teaching opportunities arise is related to the reasons for the emotional reactions manifested by the patient. Perhaps a certain patient is extremely irritable and often critical of everything done for him. During the discussion, reference is made to the fact that "He is an old crab," or "You can't please him no matter what you do." This is your signal that the group needs some teaching to increase their understanding of a specific need or reason for the particular behavior of this patient. When they understand why the patient reacts as he does, you can plan together an approach that will help the patient. Perhaps you decide that this is his way of "getting even" with the hospital routines, which regulate his every move and allow him nothing whatsoever to say. Asking him to choose between two different times for the giving of certain care or consulting him about how he wants his room arranged may be all that is necessary to make him more cheerful and cooperative.

Perhaps at this point something should be said about questions asked by your staff. As a rule, you should always encourage them to ask questions. This does not mean that you will answer every question. Remember that you cannot allow the discussion to be sidetracked from the patient. You may have to tell the person that a particular question cannot be considered at this time. If a question is asked that you feel they, or at least one of them, should be able to answer, hand it back to the group. Make them do a little thinking. On the other hand, a question may arise which is actually beyond the understanding of the group. It is at this point that many leaders get panicky. Here are some suggestions to help you if you experience this reaction:

1. Whenever possible, answer the question, using simple terms and not too much detail.
2. If you don't know the answer, do not try to bluff. Tell your group frankly that you do not know. You will gain much more respect from them. Then plan to find the answer. You may ask someone in the group to look up the information, or you may indicate that you will find it and tell them at the next conference. Then keep your promise.

EVALUATE AND SUMMARIZE. You are a listener as your staff brings out their thoughts and observations. You must evaluate all that is said and sift out that which is important for the good of the patient. They may not always realize the significance of what the patient said or of what they see. You are the one who will make use of this information. No item is too small to be considered since it may be the final clue needed to determine the nursing care that the patient should have.

RECORD PROBLEMS AND APPROACHES AS EACH IS DECIDED UPON. As the conference progresses, you should record on the nursing care plan those problems and approaches you have helped your group to recognize. Do not try to identify any set number of problems for every patient. One patient may have only one problem, whereas another may have two, and still another may have four or five areas in which plans for specific nursing care must be made. The main thing is to consider the *total* needs of the patient. Then select one or two main problems. It is better to identify and solve one real problem than to look for many problems and offer only superficial suggestions for their solution.

DETERMINE AND RECORD THE AIM OF NURSING CARE. After making a nursing diagnosis, i.e., identifying patient needs and nursing problems, you must determine the over-all objective or aim of care for the patient. This aim arises from, or is based upon, the needs and approaches already recorded or upon the aim of therapy planned by the doctor. Although general in form, it cannot be made too general. For example, wording the objective this way, "To help the patient get well," is a general aim, which is true for every patient in the hospital. It must be made more specific. Frequently determining the aim or aims of nursing care, i.e., what is to be accomplished for the patient or what you will help him accomplish for himself, must come before deciding on the specific nursing measures which can be used to reach those aims.

USE THE INFORMATION FROM THE NURSING CARE PLAN. The conference and resulting plan of care will benefit the patient only if the information is used. Refer to the care plan when making out assignments and when giving or receiving reports. Use it as a guide when giving nursing care. Show your staff how to use the plans. Gradually, you will find everyone depending more and more on them for information concerning how to care for their patients. As a result, the functional approach to nursing care will be eliminated and everyone—patients and workers alike—will be happier and more satisfied.

Close the conference on time even though the group is still interested in further discussion. Under no circumstances allow the conference to "drag" even if the allotted time has not been used. By closing while interest is still high, you are preparing for the next conference.

Maintaining Group Control During the Conference. Every group is made up of individuals. If you can control each person and help her to make satisfactory contributions to the general discussion, you will have few problems in controlling the group as a whole. A number of general suggestions have already been made to help you guide the discussion. Here are a few additional suggestions concerning individual and group control:

THE PERSON WHO TALKS TOO MUCH. This individual is always ready to answer at some length any question you may ask. Often she will include unnecessary information. You may use any one of several techniques to control her participation and to give others the opportunity to express their ideas. You may look at your watch, wait for the end of a sentence, then interrupt her and thank her for her contribution; then suggest that you want to hear the opinions of someone else or ask what point is being made. When you ask a question of her, word it so that she needs to answer either "Yes" or "No." Sometimes you will have to ignore her when she indicates that she wishes to talk. This individual may, however, do most of the talking because she actually knows more than the rest of the group; therefore, they rely on her to provide the necessary information. In that case, try to draw out the others first, then use this person to summarize or to give additional information.

THE PERSON WHO TALKS TOO LITTLE. There are usually one or two such people in every group. They may be bored, uninterested, or shy. If possible, determine the reason for their lack of contribution. Find something of interest to the person and ask her to talk about it. If the individual is afraid to speak in front of a group, give her a chance to prepare, by asking her to find out beforehand some specific information about the patient; then ask for her experience or information. Usually it is necessary to call on this person directly. Always thank her for her contribution when she has finished.

PERSONS CARRYING ON A PRIVATE CONVERSATION. Keep the discussion moving fast enough so that everyone will have to listen in order to keep up with the ideas being offered. When you notice a private conversation in progress, pause and let the others listen. You may also ask these people to give their information to the entire group. Another way of breaking in is to ask a direct question of the one who is doing most of the talking.

CONTROLLING AN ANTAGONISTIC GROUP.   Occasionally, you may sense a feeling of antagonism within the group during a conference. If possible, discover the cause. Get the antagonistic persons to talk about their work. If their antagonism is caused by a lack of information or a misunderstanding, try to correct this condition immediately. The group must be able to work together cooperatively if they are to plan good nursing care. Avoid seeming to "push" them. Use those who seem more responsive to help change the feelings of the others. Praise them whenever possible. If you feel that one person is responsible for the attitude of the group as a whole, you may need to have a private conference with her in an effort to clear up her antagonism.

CONTROLLING A PASSIVE GROUP.   To encourage participation, discover some point of interest and get passive people to talk about that; however, avoid allowing one or two of the group to do all of the talking. Use more illustrations. Ask simple leading questions. Give additional praise for participation.

CONTROLLING AN ACTIVE GROUP.   The group who thinks quickly and participates readily and actively presents a great challenge. Keep ahead of them, moving quickly from point to point. Avoid superficial consideration of the problem under consideration. Use more difficult questions, thus encouraging the group to give more thought to the subject being discussed. Keep the discussion patient-centered.

The conference gives you the opportunity to know your staff better and to weld them into an integrated group capable of working together harmoniously and cooperatively. Your success as a conference leader will enhance your leadership in your job.

QUESTIONS ASKED ABOUT THE NURSING CONFERENCE

Why is a conference necessary? The conference is the only practical means whereby everyone's ideas, observations, and suggestions about the patient and his care can be combined and the best ones selected. When you recognize the wealth of information that your staff have about the patients, you will want to make use of it whenever possible. Unless all of you work together toward a common goal, you do not have teamwork. The leader who "bosses" those who "work for" her does not exert true leadership. The conference helps every person to feel that she has a responsibility toward the patient, because she helped in the planning of his care. Unless your group meet together to discuss and plan the nursing care for each patient, you and your patient will miss the benefit of their ideas.

How can I find time for the conference? This depends upon how strongly you want to hold the conference. If you are really convinced that the conference is necessary, then you will find the time. Review the day's program, then select a time when there seem to be fewer activities. Most people find that this occurs in the early afternoon or early evening. Now survey the situation. Do some scientific thinking, research, or problem solving as described in Chapter VI in order to determine where you can reorganize or revise the day's activities to save 10 or 15 minutes a day. Then use that time for your conference.

How personal can you make the discussion about the patient? A discussion may be as personal as is necessary to help the staff understand the patient and why he needs certain care. This is also an excellent time to review the principles of ethics concerning confidential information. I am always amazed at the amount of knowledge that the nurses' aides, and even the housekeeping workers, have about the personal lives of our patients. However, I wonder if we are helping these people to use their information correctly. On the other hand, if a patient requests your help in a confidential matter and you are able to give him the necessary assistance, you would not need to bring this information to the conference because you have already taken care of the problem.

What should be on the conference agenda? The topics you can discuss at the conference will be determined by the needs of your patients and the needs of your staff. Usually the needs of the staff are based upon, or are outgrowths of, the needs of the patients. Various topics, in addition to the planning of the nursing care for a certain patient or for a number of patients, may include questions they want answered, difficulties they have encountered in their relationships with patients, difficulties in performing certain procedures or in giving certain aspects of care, or problems in coordinating the work of several individuals, etc.

STUDY QUESTIONS

1. What are the results of the conference?
2. What methods or suggestions could you use to overcome the resistance of the staff toward spending time in a conference?
3. What are the best times for holding the nursing care planning conference?
4. What is the difference between the nursing care planning confer-

ence and the conference held at the time of the patient report and explanation of the assignments?

5. Should any member of the group other than the professional nurse be given the responsibility of leading the conference? Why?

6. Select a patient for a conference. Discuss your own preparation and that of the people who are working with you.

7. What methods can be used so that every patient will be considered at some conference and have a nursing care plan?

8. What factors need to be considered when selecting a patient for a conference?

9. Select as many methods as possible that you can use to keep the conference discussion patient-centered.

10. What incidental teaching concerning ethics could be done during the conference?

11. Discuss each responsibility of the conference leader. What techniques can be used to meet each responsibility?

12. Devise a rating scale for evaluating the effectiveness of the conference leader.

13. Should personal or confidential information about a patient be discussed during the conference? Give reasons for and against. How can you determine what information should be included and what, if any, should not be?

14. Explain briefly and in as simple terms as possible, as you would to a group of nurses' aides, each of the following:

    a. Myocardial infarction
    b. Cheyne-Stokes respiration
    c. Spinogram
    d. Auricular fibrillation
    e. Sympathectomy
    f. Atelectasis
    g. Iodine uptake test
    h. Hydronephrosis
    i. T-tube drainage
    j. Retinal detachment

Chapter 9

How to Use the Patient Care Plan in Supervision

The professional nurse must use the techniques of management and supervision to help her staff give good patient care. She must be able to provide leadership that will ensure that the patient receives the care that he needs at the time and in the way it should be given. The patient care plan lists the physician's orders and general care routines, usually called treatments and medications, and the nursing orders for nursing intervention, usually called the nursing care plan. The patient does not receive complete care unless the entire plan is used to guide the activities of the nursing staff. This section will discuss a number of ways in which the professional nurse and her coworkers can use the total patient care plan.

USE THE PATIENT CARE PLAN IN ORGANIZING YOUR WORK

Planning Is a Part of Patient Care Management. In order to accomplish anything you must first have a plan. Planning means constantly thinking ahead and deciding on a course of action. It is your responsibility to determine what must be done, who will perform the various parts of care, when, and how. You decide what care is important for the patient, and who is qualified to give that care as ordered on the nursing care plan, as well as the treatments ordered by the doctor.

KNOWLEDGE IS NECESSARY FOR GOOD PLANNING. Since part of the aim of nursing is to give patient-centered care, you must become acquainted with the patient as an individual and become

aware of his problems. You must also have the necessary knowledge
and skill to give the kind of care that his condition and problems
demand. You may have a nursing care plan already available; however, if you are just beginning to use nursing care plans, or if you
have recently admitted patients for whom care plans have not yet
been developed, you will need to visit your patients in order to get
enough information to help plan your work.

You must also know what is expected of you in performing the
duties and responsibilities of your job and what authority you have.
You will need to become familiar with existing hospital policies and
routines, both written and unwritten, and with any changes as they
are made. Various ways may be used to inform you of these policies
and changes; for example, the hospital policy book, the ward manual
(sometimes called the secretary's manual or head nurse's manual),
written memoranda posted on the bulletin board, verbal reports by
the head nurse or supervisor, or the in-service educational program.

You will need to have some definite information about the
various staff members not only about the duties to which they may
be assigned but also about their abilities and limitations as individuals. Job descriptions can usually be found in the hospital policy
book or similar manual. As you become acquainted with each person, you will gain a more complete understanding of her likes,
dislikes, aptitudes, and attitudes. When planning the work, you
should use this personal information in order to coordinate and
complement the abilities of each worker. For example, you may
assign a person who moves quickly but has a tendency to omit small
details to work with a person who moves more slowly and gives
greater attention to details. On the other hand, if there is a personality clash between two individuals, you will destroy the spirit of
teamwork and cooperation if you assign these two to work together.

PLANNING IS NECESSARY FOR EFFECTIVE ACTION.   When there is
no plan, only confusion exists. Planning implies knowing where you
are going, and it is necessary if you are to learn how to get there.
Without this knowledge, all activity will be so haphazard that little
will be accomplished. In good management of patient care, planning
and organization are essential not only to provide good nursing care
but also to promote cooperation. Organization is necessary if each
individual is to gain an understanding of what is expected of her.
With this understanding comes a feeling of greater security, essential
for job satisfaction and better job performance.

Organizing Your Own Work.   One word of caution must be
given concerning organization. Nursing care, if it is to be good, must
meet the needs of the patient—physical, emotional, spiritual, and
therapeutic. There is great danger that a work plan will become so
well organized that it consists only of therapeutic and physical care

given on a functional basis. You must always keep in mind all the aspects of nursing care needed by the patient. In other words, refer to the entire care plan when you are organizing your work for the day. The need to find out what is troubling Mr. Smith or to give Mrs. Jones a little extra TLC (tender loving care) is something difficult to assign, yet, if the patient is to receive good nursing care, the meeting of these and other needs must be planned for.

Basically, work organization is a problem of establishing priorities, that is, determining what care is most important to each patient's welfare and arranging staff activities so that each patient will receive the care he needs when he should have it. Skill in planning and organizing usually increases with experience, but you must try to improve from day to day. No one can make a set form for you to follow, but there are certain factors that, if you consider them carefully, will help you to organize your work more efficiently.

ANSWER THESE SIX QUESTIONS AS YOU ORGANIZE YOUR WORK— WHAT? WHY? WHEN? HOW? WHERE? WHO? Every work plan should show the answers to these questions if every phase of work is to be completed. Try to ask specific questions and to formulate specific answers.

At this time you should apply the principles of work improvement in order to arrange your nursing activities as efficiently as possible. To ensure individualized care for your patient your work plan must include the nursing orders for each patient as well as the procedural care necessary to carry out the physician's delegated therapy.

The questions *what* and *why* should be considered at the same time because they will help you to determine what care is most important to the patient's welfare. Which is more important, your spending a few minutes encouraging and showing Mrs. Jones how to move around more by herself or assigning someone to turn her at stated intervals? Should you be more concerned with giving the patient a bath and fresh linen or with helping him to understand what is happening to him and how he can help in his own recovery? As a professional nurse you must answer the questions *what* and *why* in order to determine nursing priorities.

Answering the *what* questions will also give you a panoramic view of all the work and nursing care that must be completed. What ward routines must be done today? What equipment and supplies are needed?

Answering the *why* questions will indicate the order in which various aspects of care should be given. Some care may need to be completed before other care can be given to the patient. If you are short of staff for the amount of work to be done (and who isn't these days?), you will find this a very important question. Consider each nursing operation, each aspect of nursing care to decide if it is really necessary. Is it necessary to give a complete bath to every patient every day? Do all baths need to be given in the morning? Must q.i.d. medications be started at 8 o'clock in the morning?

Answering the question *when* will also help in arranging the order in which care should be given, or in determining what duties may be combined to save time and steps. Plan to give the patient as much of his care as possible at one time. Conversations, carried on during the bath or a treatment, should contain more than incidental pleasantries; they should be made worth while by meeting some need of the patient.

You will need to estimate the length of time each aspect of care will take in order to avoid conflicts in the activities of the staff. For example, if you are to start an intravenous feeding after a patient has been given her morning care, you will need to know how long the worker assigned to give that care will need to complete it. Furthermore, answering these questions will help you have all equipment available when it is needed.

To answer the question *how*, you may need to refer to the hospital policy book, the procedure manual, and the patient's care plan, or you may want to do some research on your own. Is one method of arranging duties better than another? Can you save a few steps by rearranging the equipment or by changing the method of handling supplies? For instance, instead of walking back and forth between linen closet and the patients' rooms, perhaps you can devise a linen cart. Soiled linen could be placed in a linen hamper, which the worker moves with her, rather than disposing of the linen down a distant laundry chute after the care of each patient. Try to obtain all supplies and equipment at one time. Saving steps and eliminating unnecessary motions are a saving of time and energy, which can be used to give more nursing care. Time and motion studies are basically problem-solving in nature. The nurse must be ready to change her work methods, always looking for more efficient ways to decrease the quantity of work motions, and, at the same time, improving the quality of nursing care.

You must also answer the question *where*. The geographical location of care to be given will definitely affect the time necessary to complete it. The more centralized you can make a certain number of duties, the easier it will be for the worker.

The answer to the question *who* is very important. Can this duty be delegated to a nursing assistant or to a practical nurse? If so, who is best qualified to give this part of the patient's care? There are some responsibilities you cannot delegate; on the other hand, you should not think that you must give all the care. Choosing the right person for the job is important, because you must consider not only the patient and his needs, but also the worker and her needs. Part of your responsibility in the management of patient care is to help each member of your staff increase her understanding and skill in giving nursing care. They must be given the opportunity to acquire these new skills. The principles involved in making assignments to your staff will be discussed in more detail later in this chapter.

If difficulties arise as you plan your work, apply the rules for solving problems. You should also attempt to prevent difficult situations from occurring.

FORESEE POSSIBLE EMERGENCIES AND PLAN ACCORDINGLY. Since planning means thinking ahead, you must include more than the organization of duties that you know must be completed. From your experience as a nurse, you know that emergencies arise constantly no matter how well organized the hospital ward may be. For example, a patient suddenly becomes critically ill; or a new patient is admitted who requires your constant attention. Try to leave yourself and your coworkers some loopholes, so that these expected emergencies can be taken care of with a minimum amount of confusion and rearrangement of your initial plan. For example, you may have assigned extra duties that, if an emergency arises, can be omitted for that day or done at a different time. Should it become necessary, make the adjustments in the assignments. If the emergency does not develop, you have already planned how to use the time profitably by completing this additional work. If you are reasonably sure that a number of patients will be admitted, adjust the current workload of one individual and assign her to care for the new patients.

PUT YOUR PLAN IN WRITING. This plan must include more than patient assignments and the nursing care to be given, although these items will occupy a major portion. Do not trust yourself to remember all the details; write them down for future reference. Again, a set form cannot be given to fit your situation. You will need to work out your own; however, you will probably want to include, in addition to the patient care assignments, the following:

1. A list of routine ward duties to be done, e.g., clean dressing cart, check all dresser drawers for extra blankets.
2. Reminders to yourself concerning duties that require your special attention, e.g., getting special equipment ready for a doctor, observing and teaching your team members, teaching a particular patient.
3. Notations concerning help in giving bedside nursing care needed by any of your staff.
4. Questions or observations that you want to bring to the attention of the head nurse, supervisor, or doctor.
5. Incidental duties needing your attention, e.g., meetings to attend.

Preparing the Nursing Staff. Your plans must include your coworkers. You must help them recognize that nursing care is more than just performing a procedure. Interest in the patient and a desire to help him start with you and your leadership. Sometimes definite planning is necessary to encourage the staff to become more interested in a patient and in how to give him good care.

Promoting Cooperation. A leader must be able to inspire her coworkers to work together to achieve a common goal. In order to have this kind of group interaction, each worker must know what the ultimate goal is for each patient and be able to understand how her care complements that given by someone else. There should be a feeling of *our* patients rather than *your* patient and *my* patient. You must recognize that each person has something worthwhile to contribute to the welfare of each patient, and in addition, you must be able to communicate to her your appreciation of her capabilities. Helping each worker know what is expected of her and how well she is meeting those expectations will help cooperation.

Orientation Must Precede Assignment of Duties. Webster defines the word *orient* as "to set right by adjusting to facts or principles; to put into correct position or relation, to acquaint with the existing situation." Any orientation must include information concerning not only the physical set-up of the station and the hospital, but also what the person's specific duties and responsibilities are.

The method of presentation, as well as the information included, will vary according to the aim of the orientation and the needs of the individual. You may not have to orient a new employee to the ward if someone else has this responsibility; however, orientation should be continued for several days until the person becomes acquainted with the ward situation in which she is to work. Remember the individual needs to feel secure in what she is doing. The more inexperienced she is, the more she feels the need for this security. If she does not know how to obtain supplies or information, or what work standards must be met, her feeling of insecurity is increased and, as a result, she may be unable to do her work satisfactorily or to receive personal satisfaction from her work. A person can rarely remember all the information given during the planned orientation program; therefore, you must continue to give her help by repeating and adding to the information whenever she needs it.

The new employee is not the only one who needs orientation. When a worker returns from a holiday or vacation, or after her regular days off, she will need to be brought up-to-date on new patients and any changes in policy or hospital routines that have been made while she was away. Again the amount of information and the method of giving it will vary according to the experience of the person and the responsibilities she must assume.

In any orientation, but especially that of a new employee, whenever you discover an area in which she needs more understanding, you should make plans for teaching her. Perhaps she has had several years' experience in another hospital. Remember that procedures and terminology differ from place to place. For example, the early postoperative exercises may be described in one hospital as turn, cough, and breathe deeply; in another they may be abbreviated to T, C, and H. Another place may use the term, *stir-ups*, to describe the same procedure. Make sure that she is familiar with the terms commonly used on your ward. Perhaps you mention that the postoperative bed, which she is assigned to make, will need the covers fanfolded to the left side. Noting her puzzled expression, you discover that she is used to folding the covers to the foot of the bed. These may seem to be such little things to one who is familiar with them, but to a stranger they become obstacles hindering the satisfactory performance of her work. Helping her to become acquainted with the existing situation will result in a happier and more satisfied worker, one who will look up to you and think of you as a wonderful person.

Encourage everyone to ask questions. These may indicate to you those areas in which additional information is needed by the group. As you observe them working, other areas may show up. From time to time you may need to go over various procedures and routines with the entire group. New policies and procedures always mean that you must orient your staff to these changes.

USE THE PATIENT CARE PLAN AS A GUIDE IN SUPERVISION

Planning and organizing is the foundation on which effective supervision rests. Supervision includes all the activities by which management ensures that the aims of administration will be met. Activities which are an integral part of supervision in nursing are reporting, making assignments, observing, evaluating, guiding, and teaching the workers as they carry out their assignments. Nursing supervision ensures that every patient receives good care and begins with the giving of a report about every patient on the unit to every person on the nursing staff.

How to Give a Good Patient Report. A report is one form of orientation, because its purpose is to impart information about the existing situation; therefore, it is used to prepare the personnel for their day's work. Complete, concise reports are vital to good management and administration. No group can function efficiently without this method of communication. Every staff member, whether she is a graduate nurse or a nurses' aide, should have some knowledge of the patient's condition, including his problems and suggested methods for helping him, as well as of his treatment and progress. A report will give each person this information quickly.

You will have occasion to use many kinds of reports; however, at this time the emphasis will be on the patient condition report. This report is given before the staff start their work for the day and is not the nursing care conference. Any information about your patients is important to you and to every member on your staff. You must receive a report from the previous shift, and you must pass on that information to your coworkers. They, in turn, should report to you their observations, as well as their progress in caring for the patients. Their information, combined with your own observations, will then need to be relayed to the head nurse, supervisor, and oncoming personnel. This constant exchange of information is essential to make your leadership effective, and to provide good patient care.

In order to give adequate nursing care, everyone in the group must receive a report about every patient to whom she will give any kind of care. Here are some suggestions designed to make your reports more complete and helpful.

EVERY REPORT MUST BE GIVEN PROMPTLY. Other duties can be taken care of later, or someone can be assigned to care for an emergency if one exists. A delay in giving the report contributes to confusion, which in turn leads to further delay and to errors in giving necessary care. Changes in a patient's condition may alter the methods of giving his care. Each person must be informed of these changes to insure safe care for the patient. Most errors can be traced to a breakdown in communication, frequently in the giving, or not giving, of a report. Since, as a professional nurse, you are responsible for all patient care given, you are also responsible for giving them the necessary information so that they can perform their duties properly. Organized leadership demands that a thorough, concise report be given promptly at the scheduled time.

ALWAYS CALL EACH PATIENT BY NAME. Nothing destroys the individuality of a person as quickly as speaking of him as "the appy in room 4204, bed 2." He ceases to be a real person and becomes instead a disease and a bed number. Calling the patient by name not only identifies the exact person about whom you are speaking, but also helps your coworkers to think of him as an individual. Of course, you will need to include other information such as room number, doctor's name and patient's diagnosis, but these are important only because you have first identified as a real person the patient to whom they belong.

ALWAYS USE THE ENTIRE PATIENT CARE PLAN AS A GUIDE IN GIVING A COMPLETE PICTURE OF YOUR PATIENT. This plan includes the therapeutic treatment of medical problems prescribed by the doctor and delegated to the nurse. It also includes the treatment of nursing problems or patient problems as listed on the nursing care plan. Information from both areas is necessary if the patient is to receive total care. The report usually gives information concerning what has been done for the patient and how he responded, as well as what should be done and how to do it. It is very important to report how the patient responded to the suggested nursing care actions. Be sure to call the attention of your group to any changes that have occurred in the patient's condition. Report any deviation from routine methods in carrying out the physician's orders or the nursing care, e.g., specific observations to be made, topics of conversation to be avoided, or the specific time when certain care is to be given.

KEEP THE REPORT ON A PROFESSIONAL LEVEL. Avoid gossiping or saying derogatory things about any patient. Sometimes the question arises concerning how much information to include in the report to nursing assistants or in the discussions during the nursing conferences. Perhaps the best way to decide this question is to determine if the information will help the workers to understand the patient and his illness, thereby enabling them to give better nursing care. If the answer is *yes*, give them the information. Remember that the nurses' aide and the practical nurse are the ones who spend the most time with the patient; consequently, the patient may tell them more of his personal problems than we realize. It is important that they understand what the patient can and cannot do and why, so that everyone can give safe nursing care and correct information to the patient. They need to recognize, although they may not understand, the relationship between the patient's disease and his behavior. For instance, they would be more sympathetic toward the patient who has suffered a stroke if they recognize that his irritability may be a symptom, or the result, of his physical condition. Or they will be better prepared to care for the patient with multiple sclerosis if they know beforehand that the fact that this patient laughs one minute and cries the next is a manifestation of the disease and is not related to anything they have said or done.

The following incident also emphasizes the need for complete explanation of the patient's treatment. An order for "No Smoking" was left for a patient who was to have lung surgery; however, he continually begged everyone for just one cigarette. Finally, a nurses' aide, feeling sorry for him, gave him one, saying, "This little bit can't hurt you." Had the nurse explained the reason for this order and indicated what information to give to the patient, everyone would have had a better understanding of this patient and would have been better prepared to meet his demands.

Of course, giving a good report takes time; however, taking time to inform your staff through the report and explanation of their assignments will save you time later during the day as well as prevent errors in patient care. You will have to determine the best time and method to give this information.

In many hospitals the entire oncoming staff attend the report. With this method everyone hears about all the patients. Receiving this information is absolutely necessary if you expect your staff to give care safely to all patients, e.g., answering calls or passing trays at meal time. This method avoids the duplication of time and effort that occurs when only the registered nurses attend a report, and then the rest of the staff get their report later, usually about only those patients who are directly assigned to them. The more times information is relayed, especially verbally, the more chances occur when vital information may be forgotten or changed.

The problem of forgetting to relay information may be partially overcome by using a tape recorder. For example, the night nurse could tape her report about six o'clock or whenever it is convenient for her. The oncoming staff members can listen to this taped report while the night nurse is finishing the last minute care of her patients. Then she can give any additional information and observations, taping this while she talks. The day and evening nurses can add their report to the same tape and in the same way when they are ready to leave. The night nurses may then be able to follow their patients throughout the entire 24 hours.

A taped report is very helpful for those people who come later in the day, e.g., staff who come at eight or nine o'clock, or the supervisor who makes her rounds in the middle of a busy morning. If these reports are saved for a number of days, they may serve as an orientation to the patients for staff following their days off. Several hospitals have found them very helpful at a later time to prove that information was reported at a certain time.

The technique of taping reports is not difficult to learn if the nurses really want to use it. We should use as many devices and machines as possible to save time. With the increased use of data control machines we will conceivably have machines that will print out previously stored information, such as doctors' orders, patients' responses and reports, and nursing care plans. The one thing that the nurse must keep in mind when using any machine is that she is still responsible for all information she inserts into the machine and for evaluating all information which it returns to her. We must control the machines and not expect the machines to do our thinking for us, for no machine can do that.

How to Make a Good Assignment. A good report is the beginning of a good assignment. Assignments should include all routine ward duties as well as the nursing care of the patients, but avoid functional nursing when assigning the care of patients to your staff.

If they are to work together on a level above that of giving functional care, they must be concerned with more than just getting the work done. Your philosophy as a nurse is important in this respect, for you will practice what you believe. The work itself should never be considered more important than the patient or the worker. When emphasis is on the work alone, both the quality and the quantity of work decline.

You must coordinate the activities of your staff in order to provide patient-centered care. In nursing there are some areas which cannot be assigned, or at least are difficult to assign, on a functional basis; consequently, they are often omitted when that method of assignment is used. For example, how can you assign one person to give encouragement to the patient who is afraid or depressed, or to give that personal touch, sometimes called tender loving care, or to allow a patient to talk about his troubles? If you are a head nurse or a team leader, you are the only one who can insure that all needs of the patient are met. This can be done only if everyone knows what should be done for each patient and plans together how to do it. These plans must be put in writing and used when making assignments so that the patient will receive the care he needs.

COMMON MISTAKES MADE IN GIVING DIRECTIONS. If you and your coworkers are to accomplish anything, everyone must know and understand what she is to do. Here are several reasons why your directions are sometimes not carried out as you intended.

The most common mistakes are: speaking indistinctly, talking too fast, or using words not understood by the worker. When you are in a hurry, do you slur your words, or leave out words, or use abbreviations for technical terms? Do you take for granted that the person will understand what you mean? One nurse directed a nurses' aide to "check Mrs. Jones for discharge." What she meant was "for drainage"; however, the aide thought she meant to check Mrs. Jones "to go home." The rules for effective communications must be constantly observed when giving directions.

Another common mistake is giving directions in a disorganized or haphazard fashion. It is extremely difficult to remember what to do if the nurse goes back several times to include some information or direction she forgot to put in its proper place. Make sure that you know what you want the person to do and how you want her to do it, then tell her step by step. Don't rush through it; give yourself, as well as the other person, time to think about what you are saying.

Giving too many directions at one time is confusing to the person who must follow them. This is especially true if the directions are given verbally and without regard to logical order. You must consider the experience of the individual when giving her directions. The less experience she has, the simpler you must make your orders. If there are many things to do, the directions must be placed in writing to serve as a reminder and to safeguard against any omission.

Poor grammar may result in misunderstanding. The placement of words in a sentence gives meaning by indicating relationship. When placement is wrong, the exact meaning is lost. Faulty pronouns of reference are especially likely to result in such misunderstanding.

The pronouns *it, this, that, those, them* must be used carefully. For example, "Put *it* on *that* shelf over there" could be very confusing if the person did not know what *it, that shelf,* and *over there* referred to specifically. For clarity, use the exact word rather than a pronoun, or use each pronoun so that there is no question concerning its reference.

One of the biggest mistakes is assuming that your directions are understood. What seems very simple to you may appear very difficult to someone else. It is always dangerous to assume that any individual understood what you said just because you told her once. The interpretation of an idea is always based upon the listener's past learning and experience. Always make sure that each person understands exactly what she is to do and when and how to do it; for example, you may ask her to repeat your directions or you may ask her questions about how she is going to complete her assignment.

MAKING INDIVIDUAL ASSIGNMENTS.   When making out the assignments for your group, you must always consider both the patient and worker. Nor can the needs of the patient always be considered before the needs of the person who is to care for him. In order to do her best, each person must feel satisfied with her job. Here are a few suggestions designed to help you in making assignments to your individual coworkers.

Have a Thorough Knowledge of Your Job.   This is one quality your staff considers very important. They want the person leading them to be capable of giving them intelligent help and guidance. This means that you must know what nursing care is needed by your patients and the best way to give it. You must know where and how to obtain the necessary supplies, equipment, and information. You must be aware of the other duties that should be completed and recognize their relationship to the functioning of the ward as a whole. You need an over-all plan for your group and a more specific plan for your own work. You must be able to communicate effectively and to maintain good human relationships.

Consider Each Worker as an Individual.   Making out assignments is more than dividing the total number of patients by the total number of people available,° thereby assigning everyone the same number of patients to care for. An assignment, if it is to provide for good nursing care, cannot be based on number of patients only, nor is an equal division of tasks always fair if number of duties alone is

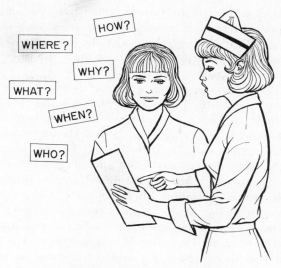

Figure 6. Directions must be complete.

considered. To make out a good assignment you should consider each worker as an individual and make her assignment based on these factors: it should be related to her previous experience; it should provide for new learning experiences or for the reinforcement of skills recently learned; it should be within her ability to complete; it should be interesting; it should provide a sense of satisfaction.

New responsibilities are always challenging and stimulating. Of course, you must make certain that each person knows how to do the work assigned to her, or, if not, plan to teach her as she works. In addition, you must follow hospital policies in assigning specific duties to the proper person.

An assignment must be fair, yet within the ability of the worker to complete it. It should be stimulating enough to make her want to learn more and to do her best. On any hospital ward there are a number of routine, somewhat boring tasks that must be done if the ward is to run smoothly. Don't give all these tasks to one person. Spread them out or combine them with new or more interesting duties. It is very unwise to take advantage of the willing worker or to show favoritism in any way. Whenever possible, rotate duties so that everyone becomes acquainted with all the patients and has a chance to learn all of the ward routines they are capable of doing.

When assigning the number of patients to be cared for by any one individual, you must consider the amount of care each patient needs and the time necessary to complete that care. You must also take into account the rate of speed with which the individual performs her work, although you cannot penalize the rest of the staff by giving one person a smaller assignment because she is a slow worker. Rather you should try to determine why she is unable to complete a usual assignment in an average length of time, then help her to do better.

Plan for Staff Development. Every person should have the opportunity to learn new things. As you plan assignments, you must provide a chance for each person to increase her knowledge about how to give good patient care. This is in addition to any in-service program the agency may be carrying on. Of course, you will be guided by the individual's capabilities and her job description.

Teaching your staff is one of your important responsibilities. This may be by formal presentation, but usually it will be an informal on-the-job type of teaching. When administration purchases new equipment or institutes new techniques for your unit, you must plan for your staff to learn about them and how to use them. For this kind of information you should have a planned presentation and practice period. Your staff must also be kept informed about new ideas or methods of giving nursing care. They will be more cooperative concerning proposed changes if they are informed about these changes in advance instead of having changes announced and then be made to comply with them without really understanding them. Whenever you answer questions giving the what, why, and how of something, you are teaching. This is one reason for giving a good explanation of assignments.

Remember that you are continually teaching, since your staff will be watching you. They will observe how you meet and talk with people, how you plan nursing care for the patients, how you organize your work. Watching how other people do things is one of the most common ways of learning.

The nursing care plan especially provides a valuable tool for teaching and orientation. When new people come to you, you can use the nursing care plan to explain your philosophy and techniques of planning and giving patient care. You can refer to these plans again and again not only to increase their knowledge about patients but also to help them learn how to assess the needs of their patients.

When people return after a day off or a vacation, the entire patient care plan provides a means of informing them about the patients. The nursing care plan will also help them see the progress the staff has made in meeting the patient's needs or in helping him solve his problems.

Provide for Individualized Nursing Care for Each Patient. Use the nursing care plan in order to meet nursing and patient problems, along with the plan for treatments and medications. You would never think of planning your work without first knowing what treatments or medications are ordered for your patients. In like manner, you, and each of your coworkers, should know what techniques have been suggested to solve the individual problems of each patient, then plan to use them.

Assignments must include information from the nursing orders as well as from the doctor's orders. Some care can be given by one person with your help to individualize it according to the needs of the patient, e.g., the best way to change the bed for a patient who is orthopneic: Other care may need two people to give it effectively and safely, e.g., turning a patient to give special back care. In this case perhaps you may want to help when this care is given because you want to observe the patient or use this opportunity to teach either the patient or your coworker. In any event the worker must know specifically to whom she can go for help, and the other person must realize that this is her contribution to the care of this patient.

Some nursing care should be assigned to every staff member, e.g., offering frequent sips of fluids to a paralyzed patient, reassuring an anxious patient by visiting him frequently and offering to help him, or visiting the patient who feels lonely. Each worker should recognize that she is responsible for the needs of every patient in some way.

Everyone should be familiar with the entire nursing care plans for patients to whom they will be giving care. This is especially important when suggested care goes beyond the use or modification of a procedure. For example, in the nursing care plan on page 103 all workers should know that they should allow the patient to make some decisions and state his opinions; thus everyone can approach the patient in the same way, ensuring continuity and similarity of nursing care and contributing to the security of the patient.

As you assign the various patients or certain aspects of their care to your staff you need to rely on your preliminary planning in which you have already determined what, when, where, how, and who. Choosing the person who is best equipped to give the patient the kind of care he needs is no small task, nor one that should be thought of lightly. Consider the skills necessary to give him good care, then choose the proper person carefully. In addition the rapport, built up between patient and worker, is important to the welfare of both.

Fix Responsibility for All Duties Clearly with No Overlapping. Again you need to refer to your own work plan to insure that all duties have been assigned to someone; however, two people should never be assigned to do the same thing, for there is danger that each will rely upon the other to perform the entire task, with the result that neither does it. A broad assignment, such as cleaning the utility room, unless it is to be done by one person, can be improved by breaking it into its separate parts, then assigning each individual certain duties.

For the same reason, two people should not be assigned to care for the same patient. If certain parts of care for this patient must be done by two people, be very specific about what each is to do. If an aide can give most of the care, perhaps a nursing student or yourself can be assigned to "help" with those specific aspects of care that she cannot perform or that require more than one person. Assigning an L.P.N. to give "medications and treatments" to those patients who receive part of their care from nurses' aides can be confusing when the aides are able to give some of the treatments but not all of them. Furthermore, there is danger that this kind of assignment may degenerate into a functional method of doing the work. When you make your assignments definite and clear-cut, you are more likely to have them completed properly. In addition, it is easier for you to determine if they have been completed, and, if not, who is responsible for failing to do so.

Arrange the Various Parts of the Assignment in Logical Order and Explain Clearly and Concisely. Depending upon the experience of the worker, you may need to indicate the best time to perform the various duties assigned to her. If a certain part of a patient's care must be completed in order to allow someone else time to do something more for that patient, you must so indicate in the assignment and call the worker's attention to it as you go over the assignment with her. Give additional explanation about terms and methods of performance whenever there is some question about whether or not the worker understands what she is to do or how to do it.

Put Assignments in Writing to Serve as a Guide While Working and to Ensure That No Part Is Omitted. Sometimes additional directions may need to be included. This is especially true for patient assignment and the special aspects of nursing care, but it may also be necessary for ward routines, such as cleaning the dressing cart or checking the linen room. Sometimes nurses note these special directions on the individual assignment sheets as they make them out. Others train their staff members to make their own notations as they listen to the report and the explanation about their duties.

We can save much time and unnecessary paperwork if we help all staff members increase their capabilities and allow them to use them. This is especially true in the areas of charting and jotting down information about their assignments.

Incidental orders or directions, given after the main assignment has been explained, may need to be put in writing, depending upon their importance. Telling an aide to take a glassful of fresh water to a patient is one thing, but telling her to give an enema, which has just been ordered by the doctor, is another. The first need not be written, the second should be, especially if the aide is unable to give the enema immediately.

Make Certain That Everyone Understands Her Assignment. If you have prepared the assignment carefully and explained it thoroughly, your coworkers should know what they are expected to do. However, never assume that they understand what you have told them. Repeat if necessary. Encourage questions. Foresee possible questions and answer them as you go along.

Anticipate and, as Much as Possible, Provide for Emergency Situations and Special Nursing Activities. A new surgical patient may start to bleed. A doctor may wish to do a lengthy examination. The x-ray department will call for a patient earlier than expected. Even the best laid plans cannot always be completed according to the original schedule. Try to prepare your staff for possible emergencies. Remember that planning means looking ahead. Every plan should be flexible enough to allow for changes if the need arises.

Observe and Evaluate the Performance of Each Person. No assignment is complete until you are satisfied that it has been performed as you intended. This includes receiving a report from each worker about her observations and methods used in giving care or difficulties which occurred as she worked with her patients. You should not, however, nag or stand over a person to insure adequate performance. Indicating your confidence in each person's ability to do good work will usually encourage each one to do her best. On the other hand, your own observations are necessary, along with a report from each person about her patients and her work, if you are to obtain a complete picture of the care each patient received. There are many methods of observation which you may choose. Some of these will be discussed later.

Your manner in giving directions is important. As a nurse, you must learn how to work and get along with people. The manner in which you give directions and explain assignments will indicate to your coworkers your attitude about them as individuals. Always keep in mind that you are working *with* them, that they are never working *for* you. The degree to which your leadership is creative, and the situation itself, will determine to a great extent the manner in which you give directions.

There are Times When You Will Need to Give a Direct Order or Command. In case of emergency or danger, when time is important, you are the only one who has the necessary knowledge; therefore, you tell each person just what to do. Sometimes in order to control certain types of individuals, e.g., the one who is lazy or indifferent, or who refuses to follow accepted procedures, you will find that the direct approach is more effective than any other.

You May Occasionally Use an Implied Direction. When your group

has learned to work together efficiently and has gained more experience, you can sometimes suggest the action that you want taken.
For example, you enter a patient's room while his care is being given
and find it somewhat cooler than you believe is safe for the patient.
You may say, "It seems rather chilly in here." The experienced
worker will get the hint. You may also use this approach to stimulate
a person to develop more initiative.

You May Want to Call for Volunteers. This is a valuable method
when a disagreeable job needs to be done, or when extra work needs
to be done. Do not allow the group to depend upon one individual's
volunteering all the time. Also you will help strengthen cooperation
if you offer to help whoever volunteers.

*The Most Common Method of Giving Directions Is by Making Them in
the Form of a Request.* There are many different ways for wording a
direction in this manner; for instance, "Will you . . . ?" or "Let's . . ."
or "How about . . . ?" This method stimulates cooperation and helps
get more work done. It works well with the person who is extremely
"touchy" or with one who is your equal in rank. It will also work with
the person who is interested in her job, or with the individual who is
older than you are and may, therefore, dislike taking orders from
you.

Your own preparation, as well as that of your individual staff
members, is important in keeping the work moving ahead smoothly.
It is during this time that you either win or lose their cooperation
and confidence for the day. Needless to say, how they feel toward
you will be reflected in the quality of nursing care they give. You
must be able to inspire their confidence in you as a leader by
displaying self-confidence but not conceit, by being firm but not
intolerant, by formulating plans that are well organized but not
rigid, by considering the needs of the individual, yet not forgetting
the welfare of the group.

How to Keep Organized. Remember that planning is a continuous process. Rarely will you be able to complete your original plan
without change. If a rearrangement of duties becomes necessary,
you need to evaluate the situation, changing as little as possible, in
order to minimize confusion and chance of error.

CARRY YOUR WORK PLAN WITH YOU AT ALL TIMES. Do not trust
your memory. Review your plan periodically to insure that nothing
is forgotten. Always refer to it before starting each part of your
assignment. Make notes on the information that needs to be recorded on the patient's chart or relayed to the head nurse or supervisor. Jot down ideas for your closer consideration about improving
the efficiency of your group. The number of reminders that you put
in writing will vary, but you will find that you will always need a few
to keep yourself organized.

HELP YOUR STAFF TO KEEP ORGANIZED.   Although you are responsible for planning and directing the work being done by your coworkers, you must also help each person to develop her ability to plan her own work. If she is to use her time to the best advantage, she must be able to organize her duties.

Give Each Person Time and Opportunity to Plan Her Work. In order to plan what she is to do, a worker must be able to answer the same six questions — what, why, when, how, where, and who. However, she will not need to answer them as completely as you did. You must give a complete patient report to every person on the nursing staff. In addition, you will need to give additional explanation concerning the individual assignments. This is especially important when several people are concerned with different aspects of care for the same patient. As a rule, most people are able to plan the sequence of their work while you give the report and explain their assignments. You may need to give additional help and suggestions concerning possible arrangements of duties to the inexperienced worker or to one who has been having difficulties in completing her usual assignment. Remember your example of good organization will help her in planning her own work.

If you have a nursing student, she should be expected, depending upon the amount of clinical experience she has had, to develop a well-organized plan and to carry out that plan satisfactorily. As the duties increase in number and the responsibilities become more demanding, some students experience difficulty in determining the relative importance of the many tasks to which they have been assigned, and they do not know where to begin. Although this is a normal situation in the process of learning, it can be quite frustrating to the student unless she is able to obtain the necessary help. You are as much responsible for the personal growth of the nursing student as you are for any other member of your group; however, the explanations you give to her should be quite complete. You may also need to discuss the situation with the clinical instructor because she is responsible for the student's learning experiences. The ability to formulate workable plans can come only through practice; therefore, the student must be given the opportunity to plan her work and be allowed sufficient time to execute it. Furthermore, she must be helped to evaluate the effectiveness of her plan and to realize how to do better next time.

Have All Necessary Supplies and Equipment Available. Having planned how she is going to do her work, the individual is anxious to begin. Nothing is more frustrating and time-consuming than looking for supplies someone has misplaced or forgotten to order. You are responsible for having all necessary equipment and supplies available when they are needed. If you wish, you may assign this duty to one of your staff before the rest of the day's work is begun. It is wise, however, to use a written list as a guide so that nothing will be omitted.

Except in Case of an Emergency, Avoid Interrupting People While They Are Working. A well-planned day should eliminate many of the reasons for taking a person away from her work to run errands or to begin some new task. Try to anticipate changes that may occur in the treatment of your patients, and forewarn your staff to expect these changes and plan accordingly. When a person is interrupted in her work, she loses not only the time needed to perform the new assignment but also the time used to pick up where she left off. Frequent interruptions are one reason why some people are unable to complete their work on time.

Encourage and Help Each Person to Improve Her Work Habits. The person must recognize those areas in which her planning was weak or the reasons why she was unable to complete her work. Help her to evaluate her plan. Suggest changes that may improve it. Help her to realize whether or not she is organized while she works. Does she remember to take all the supplies she needs when she first goes to her patient's room, or does she make several trips to pick up items she forgot? Does she save time by combining several aspects of care? If not, you will need to help her to think ahead more efficiently. Perhaps she moves slowly; you will need to analyze whether this is a personal characteristic or whether a health problem exists. Sometimes individuals are unable to complete their work on time, not because they are slow workers, but because they waste time. Perhaps they procrastinate in starting their work, or they may become sidetracked into doing some insignificant duties not directly related to the patient's care. Whatever the cause, you will need to help each one improve her habits in planning and doing her work.

EVALUATE THE EFFECTIVENESS OF YOUR PLANNING AND CARE GIVEN. You should be able to decide whether you have completed all of the day's assignment within the allotted time. Determine if your patients are satisfied with the care they received. Find out if your staff are satisfied. The information you obtain in these two areas will help to indicate the results of your plan. If certain weak areas appear, indicating that better organization could have been used, determine what was wrong with the original plan, then try to avoid these mistakes the next time.

At first this process of planning will take some time, but, with practice, you will discover how various aspects of your work fit together most efficiently. A few minutes spent in this preliminary organization will save minutes, or even hours, later in the day. In addition, much of the aimless confusion, which is a source of tension and frustration for both you and your staff, can be eliminated.

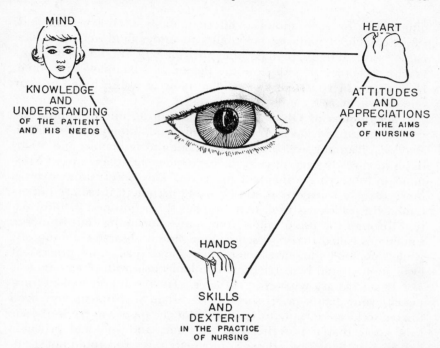

Figure 7.   Areas to be supervised. The mind and the heart must guide the hands in the practice of nursing. Adapted from Perrodin, Cecelia: Supervision of Nursing Service Personnel. The Macmillan Company, 1957.

HOW TO MAKE OBSERVATION AN IMPORTANT PART OF SUPERVISION

What Areas Should Be Observed.   Cecilia Perrodin* suggests in her book, *Supervision of Nursing Service Personnel,* that three elements are necessary in good supervision. These are the *mind,* which gives an insight into supervision and its aims and functions, the *hand,* which puts into practice the art of supervision and, last but not least, the attitudes and appreciations, which are the *heart* of supervision.

These same elements also suggest the areas that need to be observed during supervision, because the *mind* and the *heart* guide the *hand* in the giving of good nursing care, and one cannot be separated from the others. All too often concern is shown only about the correctness of detail and the manual dexterity demonstrated in the performance of care given by the individual, while little, if any, consideration seems to be given to the degree of empathy or understanding manifested by the worker for the patient. Each patient is

*Perrodin, Cecilia M.: *Supervision of Nursing Service Personnel.* The Macmillan Company, New York, 1957, page 29.

important, for each shows a different ability of the worker and, when combined, indicate her ability to understand and give total patient care. When separated, they provide only fragments of information; together they disclose the person as a complete individual. How then can you supervise so that all areas are included in your observation of each member of your staff?

Techniques of Observation. As a tool of administration, the process of supervision makes use of different, although interrelated, activities. Planning and organizing, making assignments, and teaching have already been discussed. Now comes the follow-up, which is done by observing your staff in action. This observation involves more than just inspection and checking, although these are important. Observation, as used here, implies the acquisition of information through the use of all of your senses, including your intuition, sometimes called the sixth sense. You should observe continuously, while you look, do, talk, listen, write, and read. The process of evaluation should be carried on simultaneously with observation.

LEARN TO SEE WHAT YOU LOOK AT. Have you ever looked for a pencil, your bandage scissors, or a certain instrument and been unable to locate it, only to have it suddenly appear in front of you? You know that it was there all the time, and you had probably looked at it many times during your search, yet you could not see it. This can happen to you also as your observe your staff. However, through conscious effort, you can increase your ability to see. Here are some suggestions that may help you learn to see what you look at.

Have Some Idea What to Look for Before You Begin Your Observation. In order to do this, you will need to use all the knowledge you have gained in your entire classroom and clinical experience. Ask yourself continuously what and how, for example:

1. What symptoms should I look for in this patient?
2. What safety measures should be used for this patient? Are they being used?
3. How should the patient's environment appear when his care has been completed?
4. What is each person doing at this moment?
5. Is the nurses' aide turning the patient often enough? What method is she using?

Be careful to look at every aspect of the patient's care and environment; this will include the care he is receiving and has already received. However, do not concentrate on single details only and thus neglect to obtain an over-all picture of the patient's care and his response to it. Keep in mind other information that can be obtained through what you see, for example, the sympathy shown toward the patient, or the method of adapting the principles of a procedure to fit a particular need of a patient, thereby indicating an understanding and appreciation of the patient's problems by the worker. Keep checking back on the questions you want answered, although you do not want to limit yourself to that information only.

Consider Each Person as an Individual. If you are to determine what to observe in the care of a patient, you will need to give some thought to his individual needs. When you observe someone at work, you will need to compare the care she is giving with that which she is capable of giving. In like manner, you will need to consider her attitudes, her emotions, and her differences. It is impossible to pour everyone into the same mold by expecting them to think alike, to act alike, or to give nursing care in exactly the same way. Your understanding of the individual should give you more self-confidence in your personal relations with her. Furthermore, a greater spirit of cooperation follows the consideration of the personal desires, needs, and abilities of the individual.

Try to Be Objective About What You See. If ten people observe a certain incident and then try to describe it, there will probably be ten different versions. Everyone will have his own interpretation of the incident and is sure in his own mind that he saw it happen that way. There are several reasons why it is sometimes difficult to get a factual account of any incident.

First of all, a person fails to be objective in his observations because his attitudes and motives may cause him unconsciously to overlook or to exaggerate certain things. It is not uncommon for a person to see only what he wants to see. It may be extremely difficult for an individual to be entirely objective when observing someone whom he either likes or dislikes intensely. Since what the individual believes he sees is often controlled by his preconceived ideas, beliefs, or emotions about the situation in general, he may generalize and then look for examples to prove that he is correct. For example, if a person believes that all teen-agers are juvenile delinquents, he will see only those incidents that tend to support his belief. He will either fail to look for or to recognize anything contrary to his belief.

Another reason for this lack in objectivity lies in the fact that a person's mind tends to supply that part of the action which he did not see, thus making those facts which he did observe meaningful to him. For instance, as a nurse passes the door of a patient's room she hears a noise and turns in time to see the patient pulling himself up into a chair from a kneeling position on the floor. Unless she is aware of the legal implications, she will probably say that the patient fell out of bed. Yet, when she is asked, she will be unable to say truthfully that she saw the actual fall. Her belief that he fell stems from the fact that she filled in an action that might have caused the noise she heard, and which would have accounted for the position of the patient when she first saw him.

When a person realizes the importance of being objective in his observations, he will also realize that he must obtain all the facts before he is justified in drawing any conclusion. Assuming that something has happened or that something is true without first obtaining substantiating evidence invalidates any conclusion based on those assumptions. Conclusions should be made only after all the facts have been collected.

You must try to be accurate and objective in your observations of both your patients and your staff. Try to obtain all the facts. For example, you should be careful in believing that a person did not do a certain part of her assignment simply because she has been known to omit it in the past. On the other hand, you are not justified in thinking that someone has completed her work simply because she has always done so in the past. You must have sufficient evidence before drawing any conclusions. The fact that a person neglected on one day to tell you about the symptoms of one of the patients does not justify your saying that she usually fails to observe symptoms accurately, that she usually forgets to report them, or, as is so often the remark if this person is a nursing student, that she does not assume responsibility.

The knowledge that your attitudes and emotions are likely to color what you see should make you especially careful in making your observations. When you feel irritable and tired, you are likely to pick up those incidents that provoke you; when you feel happy, you will tend to overlook these same incidents.

Look for Relationships or Associations Between What You See and What the Over-all Situation Appears to Be. Any incident is made up of a number of separate actions, each of which could have a number of different meanings when separated from the total incident. Therefore, it is necessary to observe not only individual steps of nursing care but also to consider each step in relation to total care needed by the patient. Do not look for errors only, but consider the entire performance of the worker. Seeing how all aspects of care fit together will indicate, to some extent, the understanding that the worker has concerning the needs of her patient. You should determine if each part of the care is correctly given, but you should also observe whether the proper sequence of steps or procedures is used.

Be Interested in What You See. Interest helps you to be more complete and accurate in your observation of details. This can be demonstrated in your ability to recognize a person and remember his name. If, at the time of your introduction to this person, you were extremely interested in him and anxious to meet him, you will later be able to describe him quite accurately and will be able to recognize him the next time that you see him. If, however, you were busy thinking of other things and gave only superficial attention at the time of the introduction, you will find it extremely difficult to remember specific details about the individual, because you did not really see those details in the first place.

Interest in your patients and in the nursing care given by your staff will increase your ability to see what they are doing, because you will tend to give greater attention to the details of their work. Concentration while consciously looking for details will also help you to see better. You can never allow yourself to become so engrossed in your own work and in your own problems that you look at, but are unable to see, the work and problems of others.

LEARN TO LISTEN. Perhaps the biggest obstacles to effective leadership lie in talking too much and forgetting to listen. Learn to listen to what others are saying. This includes listening for what is not said. People tend to omit those ideas which make them uncomfortable or about which they think they will be criticized. Group feeling is stimulated when each member feels free to offer suggestions, knowing that you will give them thoughtful consideration. Remember that your position as leader does not give you the right to do all the planning, make all the suggestions, or issue only commands. Resentment is usually the end result of such autocratic leadership, and instead of welcoming your supervision, the worker will tend to avoid it and you, whenever possible.

Some of the aspects of listening were discussed in the section on communication. As a reminder, however, remember that you need to listen for the "overtones" in a person's conversation. It is not always what is said that counts. Listen with your eyes. The tone or inflection of voice along with the facial expressions are important in giving meaning to the spoken words. Look at the person while she is speaking. Give her time to express herself and indicate your interest in what she is saying. Listen as she talks with the other workers or with her patients. Ask yourself if the information she is giving is correct, if she is displaying the proper understanding of the patient and of the care he needs, and if she shows an appreciation of his problems.

Every nurse must spend time with her patients—looking and listening. All too often nurse-patient communication is nurse-directed. Commonly it consists of comments about the weather—past, present, and future—or the casually asked question, "How are you this morning?" Directions and information are given in the same offhand manner, and the patient feels that the nurse is not interested in him personally. Most conversations can be patient-directed, although there are times when the nurse may need to steer the conversation toward definite subjects. The patient should always be allowed to choose the topic of conversation; the nurse merely helps him to express or identify his feelings. She indicates her interest without showing judgmental attitudes, e.g., disapproval, and without making decisions for him. She gives information when necessary or may offer suggestions, when these seem needed, to help the patient solve his problem. But whatever the trend of the conversation, the nurse cannot ignore what the patient wants to talk about.

LEARN TO USE YOUR OTHER SENSES. While your sense of taste may play a minor part in your observations, you should learn to use your senses of smell and touch to add to your information about the care your patients need or are receiving. Are there unpleasant odors? What can be done about getting rid of them? Is this patient particularly sensitive to odors? Do certain odors convey pleasant or unpleasant ideas to the patient? For example, the odor of certain flowers reminded one patient of the death and funeral of his wife and caused him to become very depressed. Does the foundation of the bed look smooth, but more than that, does it feel smooth? Is the temperature of the room or of the bath water too warm or too cool for the patient? With practice you will find many other areas for using your senses of touch and smell.

CULTIVATE YOUR INTUITION. This sixth sense comes with experience. You get a certain feeling, nothing definite, nothing that is the result of a logical thought process. It is the result of the knowledge and understanding you have accumulated from your various experiences in similar situations. While you cannot rely upon your intuition alone, you cannot ignore its presence. Perhaps the thought occurs that you should check on a certain patient. Do so; it could be important. Something tells you that not all the pertinent information has been given about a certain situation; keep searching until you are satisfied.

OBSERVE CONTINUOUSLY. Although you should observe your staff constantly, you do not want to watch any one individual too closely. Constant observation is not necessarily close observation. The first gives the worker a sense of confidence and security; the other indicates your lack of confidence and trust in her ability to do her work. The purpose of observation is to give you a source of information that you can use to guide, help, and encourage your staff in their work. Observation is also necessary to determine the effectiveness of the nursing care given.

Of course, good observation can be done only when you know what to look for and how to see it. This means, as discussed previously, an adequate knowledge of the needs both of your patients and of your group, then an evaluation of what you see in order to determine how well the needs of both are being met. This knowledge can come only through personal contact with your patients and with your coworkers, during which you consciously make use of all the techniques of observation.

Observe as You Care for Your Patients. One of the best times to observe your patient is during the time you are giving some of his care. Good rapport can be established at this time because he feels that you are doing something for him and, therefore, are interested in his welfare. Yet, how often have you seen a nurse enter a patient's room, carrying a trayful of medications, without seeming to give a thought to the patient himself? As she approaches the patient, she is busy checking the patient's name on the medicine card and the number of medicines she is to give him. When she reaches his bedside, she speaks his name or uses other means of identification, casually glancing at the patient as she does so. Perhaps she gives a word or two of instruction. Then, as she hands him the medicine and waits for him to take it, she looks again at her tray of medicines. She may glance once more at the patient, but chances are that she is thinking about the next patient rather than the one beside her. In such a situation, how much did the nurse see, hear, or feel about the patient and his environment?

As you do your work, learn to see your patient. Give your conscious attention to his expression, his color, his position in bed, his topics of conversation, and his environment. Compare what you expect to find with what you actually observe. In what aspects do differences appear? Are these differences significant to the patient's condition and to his general welfare?

Observe as You Work With Your Staff. It is generally unwise to stand by doing nothing except watching the person at work. This method of observation is the one that has caused the general belief that supervision is inspection. An opportune time to observe your staff members is during the time you can work with one or more of them in caring for a particular patient. At this time, you can observe manual skills and ability to adapt steps of care to fit the patient's needs, as well as skill in communicating with the patient and his family. You should note whether the person attends to all the details of nursing care or omits some that she may feel are not important. Her attitude toward the patient may be manifested in her approach and manner toward him or in the way in which she gives the care itself.

Observe During Your Rounds to Visit Patients. During your morning rounds, you can gather some important information as you go from bedside to bedside; however, you will probably find it difficult to gain adequate information about personal problems because of lack of time. When you visit your patients at other times during the day, try to spend more time listening to them. One of the topics of conversation may be concerned with how the patient feels about the care he is receiving or about those who care for him.

The patient's evaluation of his care is important for two reasons.

First, you are concerned with finding out how well your staff is meeting the needs of each patient, and secondly, you may find areas in which the patient complains of a lack of care or is dissatisfied with his care. Public relations is one of your responsibilities, especially those public relations that begin with the care of the patient. As Monroe M. Title* comments in his article, *Public Relations Begin with the Patient:* "One dissatisfied, misinformed patient with an average number of friends can do much to injure the reputation and the good will of a hospital."

Much of the criticism of nurses and nursing care today arises because the patients and their friends and relatives do not understand the reasons for the care given or not given. For instance, people often think that getting up on the day of, or the day after, surgery is cruel. Usually they believe that the patient is permitted to get up early, allowed to go to the bathroom, and encouraged to give certain parts of his own care so that the hospital personnel will not have to do so much work. When the patient has this attitude, the aim of early ambulation may have been achieved, but the good will and respect of the patient have been lost. Actually, this criticism indicates the need for better communication and teaching in order to give the patient a better understanding, thereby gaining his active cooperation with the activities used to aid in his recovery.

Observe as You Do Your Own Work.   Learn to weave your observation among and around your own duties. As you circulate or as you work, you have a chance unobtrusively to observe your staff at work. Avoid giving the impression that you are snooping. However, you should be able to see how they are progressing with their individual assignments, what they are discussing with their patients and coworkers, their correctness in following established procedures and, perhaps, how they display their understanding of the patient.

Observe During the Report.   The report that each person gives you at the completion of her assignment is a good source of information, not only about the patient and what was done for him but also about the attitudes and understanding of the person who gave that care. For example, when you get a report, you find out if all the work has been finished; at the same time, you can determine the worker's ability to follow directions and her interest in details. If the person is allowed to chart, still another source of information is available, for again you may find indications of the kind of work she does, whether it is hurried, slipshod, meticulous, neat, and so on. The spelling and content of her charting will also give you some idea

---

*Title, Monroe M.: *Public Relations Begin with the Patient.* Hospital Management, September, 1960, page 36.

about her interest in accuracy and the importance she attaches to this responsibility.

Observe After All Care Has Been Given. You can continue to gain information if you visit the patients after their care has been completed. Suppose you enter the room of a patient who is suffering from heart decompensation and is on strict bed rest. You see that the window shade is arranged so that the morning sun shines in the patient's face. The patient himself is sitting up on the back rest, but the pillows are arranged so that his head is pushed forward onto his chest and his shoulders are hunched foward. His arms are lying outside the bed covers, which are pulled tightly across his chest, making it even more difficult for him to breathe. In addition, the sheet and spread hang unevenly down one side. The bedside table is pushed away from the bed. The water glass is half full of water that feels warm and looks stale. The signal cord is tucked under the pillow in such a way that the patient would have to exert himself to find it.

Contrast that picture with one you observe as you enter another room. This patient, a woman with far advanced cancer, is also sitting up in bed. Body alignment is good with the head, neck, and shoulders well-supported by pillows that are arranged correctly. The patient's hair is combed and tied with a bright ribbon. There is even a hint of lipstick and rouge. The bed covers are neat and arranged to give ample movement of the feet. The shades are fixed to give plenty of light and yet shut out any glare. On the over-the-bed table are fresh water, an open magazine, and a box of Kleenex. A paper bag for soiled tissues is pinned within easy reach of the patient. The signal cord is fastened so that the patient can reach it without turning. The tube from the retention catheter has plenty of slack yet is so arranged that the fluid will drain easily into a container.

It is obvious from these observations that you can get a great amount of information about the kind of care given to these two patients, You should not, however, render judgment on what you see only. Especially in the first case you should discuss with the worker what you observed and try to determine if there are valid reasons for the apparent poor care. You should also ask yourself some critical questions about your methods of making assignments and the amount of help given to the person who was assigned to care for this patient. Perhaps her assignment was too large for her ability to complete it, or she was interrupted too many times, or she was too inexperienced to care for this very ill patient.

Whenever you are observing, remember to consider what you can learn about the knowledge, understanding, and attitudes of those who are giving the nursing care.

HOW TO USE THE INFORMATION OBTAINED THROUGH OBSERVATION

In supervision, evaluation, like observation, must be a continuous process. All information obtained from your observation must be used to evaluate yourself and your staff and to help each person to improve.

Evaluate Your Own Leadership and Supervision. Every leader must be able to criticize herself objectively and honestly, for until she is able to use self-criticism, she has no right to criticize others. She must be able and willing to improve herself, rather than offering excuses for her apparent weaknesses. Here are some examples of questions that may help in this self-evaluation:

1. Does your group accept your leadership?
2. Do you lead or do you "boss"?
3. Do they welcome your help or do they seem to consider it interference?
4. How well are you helping your group to understand the meaning of good nursing care? Do areas appear where teaching is needed?
5. Are they able to follow your directions? How clear and specific are your directions? Do you include all the necessary information?
6. Are your assignments well-planned? Are you using the individual abilities of each person to the fullest extent?
7. Are you meeting the needs of the individual worker for recognition and security? Are you more concerned with the work or with the worker?

Evaluate the Understanding, Attitudes, and Performance of Your Staff. If supervision is to be effective, you must use all the techniques of supervision, including evaluation of the work of each member of your staff. If manual dexterity and correctness in doing procedures are the only aspects considered, you will be unable to help the worker to develop as an individual. Nursing care is more than the performance of procedures. Nursing care depends upon the relationship of nurse to patient; therefore, everyone must try to improve in the area of human relations in order to increase skill in getting along with people. Here are some examples of questions that will help in the evaluation of your staff.

1. Are they able to plan their work and complete their assignments?
2. Do they understand what is expected of them?
3. In what areas do they need to learn more?
4. How well do they follow procedures?
5. Do they tend to waste time and energy in any way? If so, why?

6. How does each person get along with the other workers? Does she prefer to work alone or with someone else?
7. What attitudes do they express about their patients?
8. Are the patients receiving good care? Are they satisfied with their care?

Evaluate the Group as a Whole. Every group is made up of individuals; however, when there is a strong spirit of teamwork, the individuals cease to function independently and work together as one. Here are some examples of questions to help you to determine the effectiveness of the group as a unit:

1. Do the members of the group work together harmoniously?
2. Is the nursing care coordinated to meet the needs of the patient?
3. Is the group satisfied when their work is completed?
4. Do they share in the planning of patient care? Does each one participate in group activities?
5. Do they express group consciousness through the use of the words, *we* and *our?*
6. Do they look to you for leadership?

Help the Individual To Improve. If you are unable to help the person at the time of your observation, make a record of what you observed so that you can use it later in a conference with her. A written record concerning some observation about the person herself or about her work is called an *anecdotal note.* In some situations you, as a staff nurse or head nurse, may be asked to keep anecdotal notes on your group to help in the evaluation of the progress of the individual. It is not within the realm of this book to discuss in what job categories this responsibility should be placed. However, since you may need to make these notes, a brief discussion of the elements necessary in a good anecdotal note will be included at this point.

ANECDOTAL NOTES MUST CONTAIN ONLY FACTUAL INFORMATION. Since an anecdotal note is a written record of an observation, all that has been said about making objective and accurate observations is true of the written record also. You must try to eliminate your feelings, interpretations, and evaluations as much as possible. One of the best ways to become objective in the recording of your observations is to answer the questions, "Who did it? What was done? To whom? And when?" In other words, include only what you saw or heard, so that when you talk with the individual later, you can give specific examples of her behavior or work.

A note which states, "Miss M. gave good nursing care this morning," is inadequate. This is an interpretation by the writer and the head nurse or supervisor who tries to summarize a number of such anecdotal notes will be unable to make her own evaluation of the performance of Miss M. Such a note may not be questioned since it indicates a good performance. But suppose the note reads, "Miss M. does not seem to understand children." Immediately, Miss M. will ask, "What makes you say that?" If the specific incident that caused this remark has not been included in the anecdotal note, the person doing the counseling will be unable to help Miss M. realize why she gives this impression. Instead of helping the person, such a note will only arouse her resentment.

OTHER INFORMATION IS NECESSARY TO COMPLETE THE NOTE. The date of the observation, and sometimes the specific time of the day, should be given in order to help the individual to recall the incident. The name of the person who was observed and the one who did the observing must also be included. Occasionally, to help the person doing the final summary or interpretation, the background of the incident can be given. For example, the fact that a large assignment was completed is not too significant in itself, but it does become important if all details of care were attended to even though the assignment included a number of very ill patients. Also the completion of such an assignment would be significant if the individual was usually unable to finish her work.

A SUFFICIENT NUMBER OF ANECDOTAL NOTES MUST BE AVAILABLE TO DETERMINE THE CHARACTERISTIC BEHAVIOR OF AN INDIVIDUAL. It is impossible to generalize on the basis of a single observation. The aim of anecdotal notes is to give an accurate composite picture of the individual, her skills, attitudes, and degree of understanding. In order to attain this, no incident is too small or too insignificant to be omitted from the record.

The fact that the worker went ahead and took afternoon temperatures without being reminded becomes important when other notes indicate that she took the initiative in emptying the linen hampers, straightening the service room, and so on. The fact that a person was very abrupt in answering the requests of a patient, or looked and spoke crossly, indicates her attitude or her emotions on one particular day only. Probably one of the main complaints made by personnel, especially by nursing students, about evaluation reports is the one, "How does she know how I usually do my work? She saw me only once." For this reason, an adequate number of good anecdotal notes is necessary. Characteristic behavior cannot be determined after seeing the individual do something one time only. A number of observations indicating similar behavior are necessary before the typical behavior of an individual can be determined.

ANECDOTAL NOTES MUST INCLUDE OBSERVATIONS OF BOTH THE STRONG AND WEAK ATTRIBUTES OF THE PERSON. All too often the only notations recorded are those that indicate what the worker did wrong. To be fair, an evaluation must show the strong points of the person as well as her weak areas. This means that the recorded observations must include this information. When the person is constantly criticized for her errors, and is given no indication that her work is satisfactory in any respect, she soon loses all interest in trying to improve. Giving recognition for good work is just as necessary, when helping a person to improve, as calling her attention to those areas in which she could do better.

You may not be the one to do counseling according to its usual definition. However, since one of your responsibilities in supervision of people is guiding and helping them, you will probably need to use some of the techniques of counseling as you work with them.

Every person has the right to know how she is doing. When she is kept informed of her progress, she is better able to realize what she should do to improve. Sometimes the information you obtain during your observation will need to be used immediately; sometimes the matter can be taken care of later. Whatever the time, you should take the person aside so that you can talk privately, especially if a reprimand or correction is necessary. Never under any circumstances "bawl out" an individual in front of her coworkers or a patient. The average person is interested in learning how she can do her work better. She is always pleased to learn that her good points are recognized or that her work is satisfactory and appreciated. There is perhaps justification for the complaint, "The only time I find out how I am doing is after I do something wrong." A very important method of gaining the cooperation of your group is getting them to realize that you will give honest praise, as well as correction, when they deserve it.

At first, you may find it difficult to talk to anyone of your group about her work. You will find that a better feeling will exist if you praise first then offer correction afterward. It may also be easier to begin if you have some general opening sentences to use, for instance you could begin with:

"I would like to say how well you . . ."
"Some things which you do well are . . ."
"I have heard some very nice comments about your work."
"I liked the way you . . ."
"I want to let you know how much I appreciate . . ."
"Your . . . was very good (or was very well-done)."

Transitional phrases that you can use to approach your corrections and suggestions for improvement could be:

"However, I feel that . . ."
"However, I wonder about the report that . . ."
"Of course I realize that you started late (or some other extenuating circumstance) . . ."
"Now let's talk about . . ."
"There are some things that could be improved."

Throughout the discussion encourage the person to express her feelings or to offer her suggestions. You may want to say:

"What do you think about . . .?"
"Do you think there is a better way of doing it?"
"Was there a reason for your doing it this way?"
"What would you suggest?"
"Am I correct in my facts?"

At the end of the conversation encourage the individual to put the recommended changes into practice immediately. To encourage such action you may say:

"I am sure you will find it better (or easier) if you . . ."
"Suppose you try it this way next time."
"I am sure that you will do better next time."
"If it happens again and you still have trouble, I'll be glad to help you."

SUPERVISION AND HUMAN RELATIONS

Developing Good Human Relations. Interpersonal or human relations are the result of the give and take between people; they are influenced by the interchange of thoughts and ideas—in other words, by communication. When communication is satisfactory, good human relations are more likely to develop. This does not mean total agreement. It does mean, however, that each person is sincere in trying to find the best way to reach a common goal and is, therefore, willing to work with others in attaining that goal.

If you want others to communicate with you, you must communicate with them. If you want cooperation, you must be cooperative. If you want respect, you must give respect. If you want to develop good human relations, you must set an example. Your recognition of the individual and her needs aids in winning her respect and loyalty. Fairness and impartiality are important in the development of good relations with other people. Keep an open mind; try to understand the other person's point of view. You should strive to win the respect of your group, not because of your title but because of your desire to help them to do the kind of work they can be proud of. They want to respect you not so much for the knowledge you possess but for the way in which you use it.

Each individual wants to feel that she is recognized as a person, not just a worker. You must try to meet the personal needs of each worker—her need for personal recognition, for security, for understanding, for the opportunity to use and develop her abilities, and for information about her relationship and contribution to the patients and to the hospital. Try to give each one what industry calls a "psychological pay check," i.e., the fulfillment of these needs. Sister

Mary Margarella* gives fifteen words that influence the development of human relations:
  The five most important words are, "I am proud of you."
  The next four are, "What is your opinion?"
  The next three are, "If you please."
  The next two are, "Thank you."
  The smallest word in all the world is the pronoun, I.

Getting Along with Various Kinds of People. If your leadership is to be effective, you must be able to follow as well as to lead, to have confidence in others as well as in yourself, to be more interested in giving than in receiving, to help others and to let them help you. You must be able to work with all kinds of people.

The *average worker* is often overlooked. She does her assignment adequately, does not cause trouble, and is usually dependable; consequently, you may fail to recognize this person's need for additional help.

You are responsible for helping each person with whom you work, including the one who is average. You must be able to stimulate her and assist her in developing her capabilities more fully. By so doing you will often find that an average worker can develop into a better than average, or even into a superior, worker.

The *superior worker* is sometimes neglected also because she seems capable of going ahead and of doing her work with less direction than the others. However, you cannot always assume that because a person is above average in some things, she will be above average in everything. There are always some areas where improvement can be encouraged. On the other hand, it is true that you can expect more of this person, and you should give her credit for her ability. This credit should not, however, take the form of an additional work load, but should be something that stimulates the individual to learn more, to become more skilled, or to assume more responsibility. This type of person is often bored with routine tasks; therefore, you need to plan her assignment carefully to provide the variety that will stimulate her to greater progress.

The *fast worker* is sometimes a superior worker who is able to plan more efficiently; however, this is not always true. Working too rapidly is more often the cause of errors than working too slowly; therefore, you will need to evaluate the quality of nursing care this person gives. If she omits details of care for the sake of saving time, you will need to help her to realize this weakness and show her how she can overcome it. On the other hand, if the quality of her work is

---

*Margarella, Sister Mary: *Communication: The Catalyst.* Hospital Progress, May, 1960, page 106.

good, you must show your recognition of her abilities, not by assigning more work, but rather by including in her assignment certain tasks that require more time and attention so that she becomes even more efficient.

The *slow worker* certainly needs your help. First of all, you will need to investigate to determine the reason for her slowness. Perhaps she is unable to plan her work to make the best use of her time. If this is the case, you will need to help her to learn to organize more efficiently. Sometimes the person who works slowly does so because she is of below average intelligence, which hinders thinking and planning ahead. Such an individual usually does well when assigned to routine tasks in which she can follow a procedure already developed. Perhaps there is a health problem that needs medical attention. On the other hand, she may be a person who tries to make all her work perfect, or she may be merely inexperienced and, therefore, unsure of herself.

The *perfectionist* is often an unhappy person in her job because of her frustration when unable to perform her work at the quality level she desires. She may either become disillusioned and quit, or else lose her ideals and assume a "don't care" or "so what" attitude. Neither response is desirable. Try to develop a satisfactory compromise between what she feels is the way care should be given and the way it can be given in a particular situation. This does not mean that she loses her ideals but rather that she sets her goals where she can reach them at the present time. Help her to understand what aspects of care are most important for each of her patients, then encourage her to do her best on those aspects, rather than trying to do everything for every patient.

The *inexperienced worker* needs close supervision until she gains more skill and knowledge. This help is necessary not only to insure safe nursing care but also to give her a feeling of security. You will need to plan her assignments to include both the aspects of care with which she is familiar and also new experiences, so that she will continue to learn. The speed with which you can add these new experiences will depend upon her ability to learn and gain understanding.

You may have a very *aggressive person* who may try to get everything she wants and, if thwarted, may exhibit some other form of problem behavior, such as antagonism or argument. Some authorities believe that aggressive behavior is caused by frustration. Seek to understand the person. If possible, determine the reason for this behavior. On the other hand, you cannot afford to allow her to disrupt the group. Sometimes additional attention and honest praise, without giving in to her demands, will alleviate any feelings of insecurity or hostility she may have. Sometimes it is possible to discuss the situation frankly and arrive at an acceptable conclusion. Never argue with her; stick to the facts. Firm guidance is necessary if you are to maintain control. Above all else maintain your own self-control at all times.

The *overconfident person* also needs close supervision. Overconfidence is not the same as self-confidence. The individual who is capable of doing better than average work may be self-confident because she recognizes her capabilities and limitations and will not exceed them. On the other hand, the overconfident person is often unable to recognize her lack of knowledge and understanding and will, therefore, "rush in where angels fear to tread." You will need to give additional explanation to this person concerning what she is to do and what she must not do. You should also help her to increase her understanding of the patient, including how his care is to be given and why.

PROBLEMS THAT YOU CANNOT SOLVE

The head nurse has an important responsibility. It is to her that the staff should turn for help and advice when situations develop that are beyond their ability to handle. The head nurse must also have someone to whom she can go for advice with those problems which she is unable to solve. According to the organizational lines of the agency, this person may be a supervisor or perhaps the director of nursing service.

HOW TO USE THE PATIENT CARE PLAN TO ENSURE CONTINUITY OF PATIENT CARE

The doctor's plan is individualized and patient-centered and is changed as the patient's condition changes. The nursing care plan should be just as exact and used in the same way as the doctor's plan and orders. One of the responsibilities of the professional nurse is to provide for continuity in patient care, not only by arranging hour schedules so that people are on duty to care for the patients but also by informing the staff so they know what should be done for each patient. By using the nursing orders on the nursing care plan, she can provide for continuity of individualized nursing care just as the doctor's orders provide for individualized medical therapy for his patient.

To Ensure Continuity of Care Throughout the Entire 24 Hours. The nursing care plan, like the doctor's plan, must contain orders for care during the evening and night as well as during the day. Nurses who work during these hours should refer to these directions as a guide to the care of their patients. They are also responsible for assessing their patients' needs for the evening and night hours and writing their nursing orders on the nursing care plan.

The Entire Plan Should be Transferred with the Patient When He Is Moved. We always include the doctor's orders with the patient's record when we move the patient to another patient care unit in the hospital. We should have as much respect for our nursing orders. When the staff know what nursing problems have been identified and how the patient has been cared for, they can continue with that care without making the patient wait while his needs are identified all over again. The nursing care plan could also be a valuable introduction to the patient when he is transferred to a nursing home or when a public health agency helps him with his care at home. When a patient goes to x-ray or to physiotherapy or other departments, the people involved with his care in these departments should be informed of special aspects of the patient's nursing care which they should know about. Frequently the nursing care plan could be started in the doctor's office by the nurse there, and then sent with him when he enters the hospital. We could do much to help our patients through these experiences if we would work cooperatively with all departments and agencies.

Other Uses for the Nursing Care Plan. The nursing care plan could be retained for future reference. In hospitals which readmit patients frequently over a number of years, saving the nursing care plan as a part of the permanent patient record could be valuable as an orientation to the patient when he returns, and to the possible prevention of problems that occurred previously.

Nursing service should consider periodic nursing audits, with greater emphasis on evaluating quality as well as quantity of nursing care. If the nursing care is carefully planned for each patient so that the goals of nursing care are identified and met and the patient's needs and problems are cared for, nurses have an excellent foundation on which to begin their evaluation of the nursing care they have been giving to the patient. Evaluations could be noted on the nursing care plan as illustrated on page 103, or the patient's response could be noted in nursing progress notes. In the formal nursing care audit some of the questions nurses should answer include:

Is the goal or goals we set for the patient realistic?

Are we meeting the goal or goals?

Is our nursing diagnosis correct?

Did the suggested nursing care meet the defined need or help the patient to solve his problem?

Did we prevent possible complications by foreseeing them and using appropriate preventive nursing measures?

The nursing progress note could summarize the last item on the nursing care plan on page 103 as follows:

3/18   Pt. still depressed. Thinks he is "no good." Does not talk except when absolutely necessary. Will continue to stress any improvement and encourage him to make decisions about his care. Will try to find areas of special interest.

R. M. White, R.N.

The medical diagnosis of Mrs. C. was congestive heart failure and arteriosclerosis. Every night she climbed over the side rails. Her doctor did not want a Posey belt put on her. The nurse consulted with the patient's daughter and found that the patient usually got up to go to the bathroom several times during the night when at home.

After a week the nursing progress notes summarized the patient's response as follows:

2/17   Out of bed several times during each night. Restlessness due to desire to void? Pan offered q3h or when awake. Pt. now sleeps better and does not try to get out of bed.

E. J. Potts, R.N.

Figure 8. Two sample nursing progress notes.

Was the patient satisfied with his care? Was his family satisfied? Is he being readmitted for the same condition that has brought him into the hospital previously? How effective is our teaching?

Another use for the nursing care plan that nurses should consider is summarizing it in periodic *nursing progress notes.* The doctor's progress notes include his diagnosis, observations, therapy, and his evaluation of the patient's response to this therapy. Nurses should have the same responsibility and right to make similar notations about their nursing intervention for their patients, as illustrated in Figure 8.

QUESTIONS ASKED ABOUT SUPERVISION

Why don't people do things the way they are supposed to? I wish I knew a good answer to this. Instead of generalizing, perhaps we should put the question in more personal terms. Why don't you do things the way you are supposed to? If you can answer this, then you will know why others fail. Of course, if everyone did everything correctly, there would be no problems. We must keep in mind that no one, including ourselves, is perfect; therefore, no one, again including ourselves, will do things in the proper way every time. This does not mean, however, that we can stop trying. As professional people we must supply that incentive, for ourselves as well as for others, that will enable us to improve constantly as we work toward our goal.

How can assignments be made according to the aides' abilities? According to hospital policy, nurses' aides or nursing assistants may perform certain procedures and duties. However, simply because the policy states that she can be assigned to do a certain task does not indicate her skill in performing it. If there is a very ill patient who needs skillful nursing care, you would want to assign the person who is best qualified to give this care. Furthermore, we need to consider more than just the worker's experience and dexterity. We must give some thought to her personality, interests, physical limitations, and her ability to get along with people. When she has ability but lacks a specific knowledge or skill, you will have to arrange to help her learn what is necessary.

How can I make and use nursing care plans when the older graduates criticize and laugh at me? If you have ridiculed the enthusiasm and ideals of nursing students or recent graduates by remarking, "It's all right to teach them that way but wait until they are working, they will find that those ideas just aren't practical," I hope you will realize that you are making nursing into a technical, dependent occupation rather than helping to develop it into a profession.

It is unfortunate that a nurse who wants to be considered a professional person is often opposed to trying new methods of planning and giving nursing care, offering as her excuse, "It won't work" or "we don't have time." She should at least be honest with herself and others and say, "I don't want to try it because I'm afraid I don't know how." Every registered nurse, if she wants to be considered professional, should be anxious to try, rather than undermine, any idea that could improve the care of her patients.

On the other hand, I am sure that every instructor in nursing hopes that she can instill in her students such a keen desire to give good nursing care that they will have the stamina and strength of character to give nursing care in the way they believe it should be given, in spite of criticism or ridicule. This is the only way that nursing will make any progress and outgrow the outmoded ideas that continue to strangle it as a profession.

How can I do my own work for the day and still supervise as you say I should be doing? I would first suggest that you take a very critical look at what you consider "your work." Which of those duties could be performed by a ward secretary or some other member of your staff—perhaps with some additional instruction? Don't accept the excuse that you have always done them. Policies and routines can be changed. Many nurses tend to be too fond of "paper work" and "desk work" because it gives them a nice secure feeling. They feel very threatened if someone wants to take their "security blanket" away from them. Several studies have shown that up to 70 per cent of the paper work done by nurses today could be done by someone else. Other tasks may also be reassigned to other workers.*

------

*Christman, Luther. "The Nurse Clinical Specialist." *Hosp. Progress.* Aug. 1968, pp. 14 and 24.

Perhaps a complete revision of procedure and job description needs to be done. Apply the principles of work simplification—eliminate, combine, rearrange activities, or devise a new method. I'll guarantee you can save time—if you want to. The time thus saved can then be used to meet your legal responsibility to supervise ancillary personnel.

Should an R.N. be assigned to "give meds" to all patients on a unit? There is talk of using medicine technicians for all but p.r.n. and stat medications. I do not think an R.N. needs to be assigned to the *procedure* of preparing and giving medications, especially when a qualified L.P.N. is available. What worries me most when one person is assigned to "give meds," whether that person is an R.N., L.P.N., or medicine technician, is who will assume the responsibility of evaluating the patient's need for the drug and his response to it. The "medication nurse" is too busy to do this. Too often she takes the evaluation of a nurses' aide who says, "Mrs. Jones needs something for pain." Yet these evaluations and decisions are the professional responsibility of the nurse. Almost anyone can learn to follow a procedure. In fact some hospitals which are using medicine technicians report a decrease in the incidence of medication errors as far as procedural technique is concerned; however, I am not sure that better evaluation of the patient is occurring.

STUDY QUESTIONS

1. Compare the techniques of leadership with the activities carried on during supervision.

2. Observe your own work or the work of another nurse. Select two instances of teaching. Determine how each of the four steps of teaching was carried out.

3. Check your ability to observe and remember details. Give yourself one minute in a patient's room. At the end of the allotted time, list every specific observation about the patient and his environment you can remember. Answer as many as possible of the following questions; then return to the room and check the completeness and correctness of your observations.

   a. What was the patient doing when you entered the room?
   b. What was the patient's position?
   c. What did the patient's mood appear to be?
   d. In what position were the window curtains or shades?
   e. Where was the patient's water glass? How much water was in it?
   f. How tight were the bed covers over the patient's feet?
   g. Did the light come from over the patient's left or right shoulder?
   h. Where was the signal cord?
   i. Answer the following if they apply: How many liters of oxygen was the patient receiving? How much fluid remained in the bottle of intravenous fluid? Were the drainage tubes arranged correctly?

4. Stage a highly dramatic incident in front of a group. Have each observer tell exactly what she saw. Check the results. Were there any differences in the various reports? Why did these occur?

5. Observe a worker for several days. Make anecdotal notes of your observations. Criticize each note for completeness and objectivity.

6. If you observe a person performing a procedure or giving care incorrectly and you correct her immediately, should you make an anecdotal note of the incident? Give your reasons. How will you be able to determine the progress of this person?

7. Select several situations in which a worker must be corrected. Discuss the method or methods you would use in making the necessary correction.

8. Select a problem related to work organization on your unit. Using the principles of work simplification, try to arrive at a more efficient method.

9. Observe one person as she does her work. Determine specific activities that show good work organization. Select areas that show poor organization and indicate how they can be improved.

10. Plan the individual assignments for the nursing staff on your unit. How are the individual needs of the patients assigned? How is this information given to each worker? How did you determine the sequence of activities? How is this indicated to each worker? How are the capabilities of each person utilized?

11. What are the characteristics of a good assignment?

12. Prepare a time schedule for any shift, showing the time sequence of the individual who is supervising the nursing care.

13. Discuss all the ways in which the nursing care plan can be used.

14. Do a nursing care audit on a group of patients.

15. Write nursing progress notes for a number of patients. What information should be included? What would you have to do to make this information a part of the patient's permanent record in your agency?

PART THREE BIBLIOGRAPHY

Books

Abdellah, Fay G., et al.: *Patient-Centered Approaches to Nursing.* The Macmillan Company, New York, 1960.

Byrne, Brandon: *Three Weeks to a Better Memory.* John C. Winston Company, Philadelphia, 1952.

Francis, Gloria M., and Munjas, Barbara: *Promoting Psychological Comfort.* Wm. C. Brown Company, Dubuque, Iowa, 1968.

Little, Dolores E., and Carnevali, Doris L.: *Nursing Care Planning.* J. B. Lippincott Company, Philadelphia, 1969.

Maslow, A. H.: *Motivation and Personality.* Harper and Row Publishers, Inc., New York, 1954.

Pamphlets and Journals

Bonney, Virginia, and Rothberg, June: *Nursing Diagnosis and Therapy: An Instrument for Evaluation and Measurement.* National League for Nursing, No. 20-1085, 1963.

Donovan, Helen M.: *Determining Priorities of Nursing Care.* Nurs. Outlook, *11*:1:44, Jan., 1963.

Durand, Mary, and Prince, Rosemary: *Nursing Diagnosis: Process and Decision.* Nursing Forum, *5*:4:50, 1966.

Geister, Janet M.: *Public Relations Begin at the Bedside.* Am. J. Nursing, *50*:8:463, Aug., 1950.

Geitgey, Doris A.: *Self-Pacing—A Guide to Nursing Care.* Nurs. Outlook, *17*:8:48, Aug., 1969.

Gordon, Phoebe: *Evaluation, A Tool of Nursing Service.* Am. J. Nursing, *60*:3:364, March, 1960.

Gozzi, Ethel Kontz: *We Plan Ahead What To Ask.* Nurs. Outlook, *13*:6:30, June, 1965.

Gregg, Dorothy: *Reassurance.* Am. J. Nursing, *55*:2:171, Feb., 1955.

Hay, Stella I., and Anderson, Helen C.: *Are Nurses Meeting Patients' Needs?* Am. J. Nursing, *63*:12:97, Dec., 1963.

Henderson, Virginia: *The Nature of Nursing.* Am. J. Nursing, *64*:8:62, Aug., 1964.

Interpretation of the Statements of the Code for Professional Nurses. American Nurses' Association, New York, 1968.

Kelly, Nancy Cardinal: *Nursing Care Plans.* Nurs. Outlook, *14*:5:61, May, 1966.

Kreuter, Frances Reiter: *What Is Good Nursing Care?* Nurs. Outlook, *5*:5:302, May, 1957.

Kron, Thora: *Nurses' Aides Need Clearer Directions.* Am. J. Nursing, *63*:3:118, March, 1963.

Levine, Myra Estrin: *. . . About Patient-Centered Care.* Nurs. Outlook, *15*:7:53, July, 1967.

Lewis, Lucile: *. . . About the Nursing Process — Key to Care.* Nurs. Outlook, *16*:5:26, May, 1968.

Manthey, Marie E.: *A Guide for Interviewing.* Am. J. Nursing, *67*:10:2088, Oct., 1967.

McCain, R. Faye: *Nursing By Assessment — Not Intuition.* Am. J. Nursing, *65*:4:82, April, 1965.

Melody, Mary, and Clark, Genevieve: *Walking-Planning Rounds.* Am. J. Nursing, *67*:4:771, April, 1967.

Mercadante, Lucille: *Utilization — A Vehicle for the Effective Delivery of Patient Care Services.* Minnesota Nursing Accent, Minnesota Nurses' Association, *42*:1:5, Jan., 1970.

Ramphal, Marjorie: *A Rationale for Assignments.* Am. J. Nursing, *67*:8:1630, Aug., 1967.

Ramphal, Marjorie: *Clinical Nursing Supervision.* Am. J. Nursing, *68*:9:1900, Sept., 1968.

Roth, Julius A.: *How Nurses' Aides Learn their Jobs.* Am. J. Nursing, *62*:8:54, Aug., 1962.

Rothberg, June S.: *Why Nursing Diagnosis?* Am. J. Nursing, *67*:5:1040, May, 1967.

Schwartz, Doris R.: *Toward More Precise Evaluation of Patient's Needs.* Nurs. Outlook, *13*:5:42, May, 1965.

Seward, Joan F.: *Professional Practice in a Bureaucratic Structure.* Nurs. Outlook, *17*:12:58, Dec., 1969.

Smith, Dorothy M.: *Myth and Method in Nursing Practice.* Am. J. Nursing, *64*:2:68, Feb., 1964.

Stephens, Gwen Jones: *The Time Factor.* Am. J. Nursing, *65*:5:77, May, 1965.

This I Believe . . . About Obstacles to Effective Nursing Care. Nurs. Outlook, *17*:11:34, Nov., 1969.

Title, Monroe M.: *Public Relations Begin with the Patient.* Hospital Management, *90*:3:36, Sept., 1960.

Vestal, Anne: *Problem-solving Simplified.* Hospital Progress, *41*:2:78, Feb., 1960.

Wagner, Berniece M.: *Care Plans — Right, Reasonable, and Reachable.* Am. J. Nursing, *69*:5:986, May, 1969.

Wiedenbach, Ernestine: *The Helping Art of Nursing.* Am. J. Nursing, *63*:11:54, Nov., 1963.

Yauger, Ruth Anne, and Oberlies, Betty: *"A Do-It-Yourself" Program in Supervision.* Nurs. Outlook, *15*:4:75, April, 1967.

Zimmerman, Donna Stulgis, and Gohrke, Carol: *The Goal-Directed Nursing Approach: It Does Work.* Am. J. Nursing, *70*:2:306, Feb., 1970.

PART FOUR

PATIENT CARE
MANAGEMENT AND
TEAM NURSING

The essence of leadership lies in the ability and willingness of the individual to accept responsibility—not only for his own actions but also for the actions of the people he leads.

Chapter 10

Basic Concepts in Team Nursing

Prior to the 1940's adequate numbers of registered nurses were available so that each nurse was able to give total patient care to her own patients. During World War II and the years following, many new categories of health workers came into being. Contrasted with approximately eight categories of personnel formerly on the nursing staff, the organizational chart may now list between 12 and 17 classes of workers depending on the size of the health agency. The registered nurse has assumed different and more technical duties frequently removed from the patient's bedsides, and relatively inexperienced and untrained ancillary personnel have taken over much of the direct care of the patient with a minimum of help and supervision from the registered nurse. As the numbers of registered nurses continued to dwindle, the numbers of ancillary personnel increased. Some of the problems which had their inception during the 1940's and 1950's have not only continued to exist but have been compounded during the last decade.

WHY TEAM NURSING

Problems Confronting Nursing Today.   Nursing is in a state of evolution. The pressure of striving for recognition as a profession, combined with the changes in duties, responsibilities, and changes in the attitudes of nurses themselves, have caused conflicts between nurses and auxiliary workers and a sense of frustration within the nurses themselves. Tradition has defined the practice of nursing as the direct personal care of the sick. In present-day practice, the nurse finds herself concerned more and more with technical, supervisory, and administrative duties, and is less and less able to be at the bedside of her patients. This conflict between what the professional nurse has been taught nursing to be and what she now finds herself doing is the major problem confronting nursing today.

In the light of the previous definitions of patient care, are we being fair to the nurses' aide, with her three to four weeks of on-the-job training, if we expect her to do more than follow procedures as taught? Usually she has no knowledge, or at best a limited amount, about the patient's disease and its effect on his physical, emotional, and environmental needs. Nevertheless, she is the one who spends many hours at the patient's bedside, talking with him as she works, and answering his questions. How can we be sure that the information or the nursing care so given is correct and best for the patient? The aim of her training is implied in her title—nurses' aide, one who works under the direction of a professional nurse.

Even the licensed practical nurse with her 1 year education has, for the most part, only technical training in the performance of relatively simple procedures. Although she receives a greater amount of information concerning disease conditions, she does not learn about the emotional, or even all the physical reactions of the patients. Again are we being fair to expect her to give individualized care to all patients? The stated aim of the schools of practical nursing is to train a person to work directly under the direction of a doctor or a professional nurse.

Traditionally, the head nurse has been the person who is responsible for the direction and supervision of her staff, each person being directly responsible to her. Today, in view of present conditions in many hospitals, the head nurse has no time to give more than cursory direction, help, and supervision. Under the functional method of assignment, staff nurses have only occasional personal contact with the ancillary workers, and frequently their only contact with the patients comes during the administration of medications or treatments. They do not have the authority, or the opportunity, to direct and supervise the care being given by other personnel. There is little communication among the personnel themselves, and little or no coordination between the fragments of nursing care that each person is assigned to give. The nurses' aide and practical nurse who spend the most time with the patient, talking with him, and becoming acquainted with his personal problems, are unable to make use of this information to help the patient understand his condition or to sove his problems. Nevertheless, according to Frances Kreuter, unless the patient has been so helped, nursing care has not been given.

Team Nursing Will Help Solve Some of These Problems. Team nursing was never devised to make up for an inadequate staff; however, it was devised to provide better nursing care with the available staff. The team, by working closely together, can give better care because the abilities of each team member are utilized, and all nursing care is closely guided and supervised by a professional nurse who is the team leader. Patient-centered care is implemented by the daily team conference when the entire team discusses the needs of each patient and devises ways of meeting those needs. A written nursing care plan, which is to be used by every team member, is then made and is revised as the patient's condition changes. The team leader decides what person on her team is best qualified to care for each patient. In this way the professional nurse helps all members of her team learn what is best for each patient and insures good nursing care with individual consideration for the patient's needs and problems, although she may not be the one who actually gives the care or answers the patient's questions.

Not only are there insufficient professional nurses to give bedside care, but there are also too few nurses trained in administration and supervision to fill the available positions. Some schools of nursing include one or two courses designed to help the nursing student acquire a basic knowledge of the principles of administration. Very few schools, however, offer the student a well-planned experience in learning how to apply these principles in an actual situation. Yet in many hospitals a recent graduate, or even a senior nursing student, is expected to "take charge" with little or no help from a more experienced person.

In team nursing the professional nurse, as team leader, can gain practical experience in democratic leadership by directing and supervising her team. She can learn how to work effectively with many kinds of people; how to establish and maintain good human relations; how to plan, direct, supervise, and evaluate the work of others; and how to coordinate the activities of a number of people working together. In other words, team leadership is a practical means of preparing every nurse to learn some administrative duties and to become more skilled in giving nursing care.

The Challenge of Team Leadership. Every nurse, if she believes that she belongs to a profession, must be a leader. People look to her for help and guidance, especially in those areas pertaining to health. She must have a genuine liking for people and be sincerely interested in their welfare. As a professional person she must also be active in community affairs.

Leadership in team nursing offers a special challenge to the graduate nurse for making use of all the knowledge, understanding, and skills that her education has provided. She must be able to plan, give, supervise, and evaluate nursing care; to coordinate hospital and community resources for the benefit of each patient; to make decisions wisely and calmly as the need arises; to work harmoniously and communicate effectively with all kinds of people; to seek constantly to improve in the practice of her profession; and to set an example not only as a good nurse but also as a good citizen.

Every team leader, if her leadership is to be effective, must know the basic principles of administration, supervision, guidance, and teaching and be able to apply them as she works with her team. The team leader must be able to apply the basic principles of leadership and management of nursing care which have been discussed throughout this book.

WHAT IS TEAM NURSING?

The concepts of team nursing were conceived primarily to provide non-professional nursing personnel with more help and supervision from a registered nurse so that they, with her help, could give total patient care rather than the fragmented, non-coordinated care which is given in functional assignments. The team leader has the responsibility for the management of the care of a group of patients, but she herself does not give all of the care. She delegates certain parts to her team members. However, she cannot delegate her responsibility for planning, directing, and supervising all aspects of care.

Team nursing emphasizes the position of the registered nurse as the team leader and her professional responsibilities for the care of her patients. It also adds importance to the contribution of the team members to the welfare of each patient, in the giving of direct patient care and of information about the patient during the team conference and reports, when they can help with the planning of care for their patients. The main aims of team nursing are individualized patient care and more supervision of ancillary personnel by the professional nurse, thus improving the quality of care that each patient receives.

HOW DOES TEAM NURSING AFFECT THE MANAGEMENT OF PATIENT CARE?

What Are the Basic Essentials in Team Nursing? The first essential is leadership by a registered nurse. The team leader must have sufficient knowledge and understanding to make safe decisions about patient care; furthermore, she must be willing to accept responsibility for the outcome of her decisions and for the actions of those persons who follow her directions. She must be able to supervise all the care a patient needs, whether it is simple or complex, delegated by the physician or planned as a result of her nursing diagnosis. Unfortunately, some registered nurses are not functionally capable of accepting, or are not willing to accept, this much responsibility.

The licensed practical nurse is trained to care for patients under the direction and supervision of a registered nurse or physician. In the hospital she cannot legally accept the responsibility for making all decisions about the care her patients need. The L.P.N. may take care of patients in "simple nursing situations" or assist the registered nurse in the care of those patients who present "complex nursing problems."*

If a person is unable to assume, either legally or functionally, those responsibilities demanded of a leader, assigning that person to the *position* of team leader does not provide her with the right or ability to *practice* as a team leader. This person may be very skillful in performing procedures or quite capable of organizing work, but she will usually continue to practice functional nursing instead of helping her team members meet the needs of their patients. Furthermore, she does not organize or direct her team's activities herself; instead, she follows the assignments and directions given by the head nurse or supervisor who in reality is functioning as the team leader.

To enable the team leader to provide leadership, she must be given the authority as well as the responsibility to supervise her team members. This requirement means that when the head nurse delegates leadership responsibilities to the team leader, she must also delegate the authority needed to complete those responsibilities.

Another essential in team nursing is a written *nursing* care plan which is kept up-to-date and used as a guide in the giving of *nursing* care to the patient. The orders for nursing care along with the doctor's orders for medical therapy guide the work of the team while they take care of the patient. The nursing care plans provide a means of communication which is necessary for continuity in patient care. The team leader also uses them to help her in teaching and supervising her team members.

The team plan is based upon the principles set forth previously in this book. The main differences are (1) delegation by the head nurse of the responsibilities and activities necessary in planning nursing care and in supervising those who give the care, and (2) more emphasis on helping each person—professional nurse, practical nurse, and nursing assistant—to use her capabilities to the fullest in order to provide more complete, individualized patient care.

What Are the Results of the Delegation of Duties by the Head Nurse to the Team Leader? Probably one of the more easily recognized results is found in the lines of communication. Without team nursing the head nurse gives directions, get reports, and supervises each member of her staff. Under the team plan this line of communication goes from the head nurse to the team leader to each team

---

*Statement of Functions of the Licensed Practical Nurse. American Nurses' Association. 1964.

member. The team leader plans and gives her team their assignments, gives guidance and supervision while they work, and evaluates the care that they give. Delegation of these responsibilities gives the head nurse more time to complete her own work.

When team nursing is working effectively, the group work closely together, each member knowing how her care contributes to the welfare of the patients and how it complements the care given by other team members. Since both the team and the number of patients are smaller than the number on the entire unit, the team leader finds it easier to keep informed about what is going on and to help and supervise her group as they need it. Under such circumstances the team members learn more about each patient and how to meet his needs.

One of the far-reaching results occurring with the practice of team nursing is the development of the capabilities of the team leader. She is helped to gain skills in leadership, management, and supervisory techniques and in interpersonal relationships. She is also allowed to gain more skill in assessing and meeting the needs of her patients so that they receive the direct benefit of her professional knowledge and judgment.

HOW TO START TEAM NURSING

First of all, you must have a person, or preferably several persons, who are "sold" on team nursing and who understand its principles. Many schools of nursing include this information in their curricula. Unfortunately, nursing students are not always able to see an effective practical application of its principles, so they may become disillusioned or obtain a distorted idea about the team plan. However, if nurses understand team nursing and are interested in using it, they can quickly learn ways of utilizing its concepts when they are given the opportunity.

Whenever any Change is Proposed, Some Preliminary Planning Must be Done if You Want to be Successful. In order to crystallize your thinking, some of your plans must be put in writing. Whenever possible, encourage other nurses to work with you.

Define Your Philosophy About Nursing and What You Hope to Accomplish Through Team Nursing. Setting goals is important, and goals are always influenced by your beliefs or philosophy. These must be thought through for your own group. It is impossible to copy the philosophy and goals from another institution and try to make them yours. They will not work.

Set up General Guidelines for the Practice of Team Nursing. This means reviewing, and when necessary changing, existing policies, job descriptions, procedures, and forms. In some cases new ones will have to be made. For example, you will need to set up a job description for a team leader. Other workers will be team members and their job descriptions must be changed to meet this new assignment.

Keep Everyone Informed. Remember that this process does not take place overnight, so you must keep people informed all the time. Let them have a part in the planning whenever possible. Always answer their questions.

Whenever any change is anticipated, workers become panicky and insecure. These feelings cause them to resist the changes in every way possible. The questions that every person wants answered include:

1. What is the contemplated change? In this case, what is team nursing and how does it work?
2. How will it affect me and my job? Job security as well as personal security is at stake here.
3. What will be expected of me? Do I have to learn something new? Who will help me? What will happen if I cannot do it? Personal and job security along with self-esteem and respect from others are always of concern to the worker.

Not just the nursing staff but everyone in the hospital will want to know what is going on. This includes the medical staff and the personnel in the other hospital departments. You will need to keep these people informed too.

You must be a good salesman to persuade people that (1) this method will improve the care of patients, (2) when used effectively, it will increase the job satisfaction of everyone on the nursing staff, and (3) they are capable of using its principles.

One word of caution is necessary. Keep your information and directions as simple as possible. Call everyone's attention to those principles in team nursing that they are already using. Be as specific as possible when giving them this information. Then show them how, with just a few changes, they can incorporate more of the principles of team nursing into their present practice.

Start Using the Team Method. Allow people to get a feeling of success in using the basic essentials first in a simple way. Have someone available who can answer their questions and show them how to apply the principles of team nursing. This is important. If they are unable to apply a principle or solve a problem to their satisfaction, they will revert to the old method of doing their work.

Announcing that the use of team nursing will start next Monday and leaving the staff to flounder around without help will cause it to

fail almost immediately. Furthermore, the staff will become prejudiced against it, and you will find it almost impossible to get them to
try it again. People do not like to fail.

MAKE THE GENERAL PRINCIPLES WORK
FOR YOU

Team nursing may be used throughout the entire 24 hours on
any patient unit—out-patient clinic, maternity, long-term or self-care
units. Two people can be a team when one is a registered nurse. If
the person in charge is the only registered nurse, she is the leader
whether she takes that title or not. She is legally the only one who
can assume the responsibility for making decisions or is qualified to
give total care. In many instances evenings and nights are the times
when team nursing can be practiced most effectively. The one thing
that may be different from what the staff is now doing lies in writing
down their suggestions for nursing care.

Nurses give lip service to their beliefs in patient-centered care
and in concern for the patient. However, in many cases their actions
belie their words, because if they were really concerned about their
patients, they would not deprive them of valuable care, as they do
when they refuse to pass on information about nursing care which is
needed by the patient. No nurse is with her patient 24 hours a day,
and unless she puts the directions for nursing care in writing, the
chances are very great that the patient will not receive it.

Any number of teams may be on the unit. The number of
registered nurses and other staff will determine the number and the
size of the teams. When there is only one registered nurse, there can
be only one team. If enough staff are available, two or three teams
may be used.

HOW TO IMPROVE THE PRACTICE OF TEAM
NURSING

We should realize that we will probably never reach the peak of
perfection either in the care we give our patients or in the application of the principles of team nursing. However, the amount of
improvement we are willing to make depends upon ourselves and
how much we want to improve. It especially depends upon the head
nurse, for she must encourage and help her staff to see the need as
well as find the ways for improvement.

We can always find additional ways of meeting the needs of our patients or of helping them to use as many of their health assets as possible. Increased skill in assessing patients and in using all available resources in problem-solving should be an aim of every professional nurse. She should continually strive to increase her skills in leadership, not only in the giving of nursing care but in interpersonal relationships with her coworkers and in management and supervisory skills. Finding new ways of applying the principles of team nursing provides a constant challenge to every head nurse and team leader.

QUESTIONS ASKED ABOUT THE
FUNCTIONING OF TEAM NURSING

Is it necessary to have team conferences on evenings and nights? Yes, but I believe that in many cases you are already having these conferences in an informal way. Most of the requirements for a team conference are present when two people talk about a patient and what they can do to help him in a special way and then put into practice the nursing measure they have decided upon. The only requirement that is not met is to write their suggestions on the nursing care plan.

I thought the purpose of team nursing was to provide total patient care. Don't the assignments in team nursing cause more fragmentation of care? Fragmentation of care may occur if the team leader does not use her team members properly or allow them, or help them, to do everything for the patient which they are capable of doing. This is caused by too rigid adherence to rules instead of allowing an understanding of principles and common sense to guide one in the practice of team nursing. Practice may degenerate into functional nursing even when there is a team and a designated team leader. Fragmentation of care is always present when the emphasis of the nursing assignment is put on functions, work, or procedures.

The philosophy of team nursing is that the patient must receive total patient care individualized to meet his special needs, but that care may be provided by several people instead of one person. Nursing aides or even L.P.N.'s cannot meet all the needs of the patient or perform all the nursing techniques needed to give total care. However, if a certain team member can give all the care that is needed by a patient, she certainly should be allowed to do so. The team leader is responsible for planning assignments in such a way that one person does all she can for a patient, but someone else is responsible for giving the care that she is unable to give. The team leader coordinates all such care so that no omissions or gaps occur.

STUDY QUESTIONS

1. Why was the team method of assignment originally proposed? Do you feel that these original purposes are being met as team nursing is being practiced on your unit or in your hospital? Why? Do we need team nursing or are its principles outmoded?

2. Write your goals for team nursing on your unit.

3. Apply the principles of work simplification to your present activities. Which ones show effective use of time, energy, and supplies? Which should be changed? Suggest possible ways for making your work more efficient.

4. Discuss the difference which may occur between the *title* or *position* of team leader as given by assignment and the *practice* of team leader. Can all R.N.'s function as team leaders? Why? How can they be helped? Can L.P.N.'s function as team leaders? Why?

5. Of the following arguments frequently offered against team nursing, list all the ways in which you can change the given situation or offset the given argument.
   a. Not enough staff
   b. Not enough time
   c. Too much turnover in staff or part-time staff
   d. Staff is against team nursing
   e. Staff prefers functional assignments
   f. Insistence on rigid adherence to rules and policies (Inability to see how to use general concepts)
   g. Our doctors are different

6. Select a four hour period any weekday morning and count:
   a. The number of different people who enter a selected patient's unit; also give reason.
   b. The total number of times people enter this patient's unit. (If a person comes in several times, each time is to be counted.) How does the patient feel about having so many people care for him? How can the practice of team nursing give this patient a sense of more security?

7. What makes the practice of team nursing different from the practice of functional nursing?

8. How does the patient receive total patient care under the team method of assignment?

Chapter 11

Staff Relationships and Responsibilities in Team Nursing

COOPERATION BETWEEN THE TEAMS

The spirit of cooperation, while necessary among the team members themselves, must extend beyond the boundaries of the team itself. It should permeate the atmosphere of the station, the department, and the entire hospital. If the philosophy of the team plan becomes a motivating force within each team member, then its influence will grow and expand to include all personnel within the hospital.

One of the areas where cooperation is extremely important is among the teams themselves. It is very unfortunate when one team draws an invisible line, separating their patients from those of every other team, and then refuses to step over this line for any reason. Each patient is everyone's responsibility. The fact that a patient is assigned to a particular team does not mean that only members of that team are responsible for helping that patient. The activities of all hospital personnel must center around one person — the patient — and every person in every department of the hospital must share in the responsibility of his care.

The teams must work together to insure that adequate nursing care is always available for all patients on the station. While one team receives its report and assignment, the rest of the staff must assume the responsibility of caring for the patients. In addition, the time of the conference must be selected so that another team will be free to care for the patients while the one team is planning its activities.

We must guard against the development of this invisible, yet nevertheless present, Iron Curtain which causes a person to say, "I can't answer that light because that patient isn't on my team." Every staff person has some responsibility for every patient on the unit. On further questioning the person often indicates that her real reason is that she is afraid to try to help a patient when she has not received a report about that patient. Therefore, if we expect a worker to assume any responsibility, no matter how small, for a patient, the worker has a right to know something about the person she is expected to help.

The spirit of cooperation must extend beyond a single station. There must be teamwork among all the departments within the hospital if the aim of providing good care is to be achieved. All personnel must recognize the contribution every department makes to the welfare of the patient and be willing to work cooperatively with each department to make the services of the entire hospital available to the patient.

RESPONSIBILITIES OF THE HEAD NURSE IN TEAM NURSING

The Over-all Responsibility of the Head Nurse. The head nurse is a key person not only on her station but also within the hospital. As a manager, she is responsible for all patient care given on her station and is concerned with the direction, supervision, and evaluation of that care. As part of this responsibility, she must coordinate not only the activities of her staff, but also, if there is no unit manager, all hospital services for the benefit of the patient. Since she is primarily concerned with people, she has a great responsibility in the establishment and maintenance of good human relations. The example which she sets in her day-by-day relations with her staff, with other hospital personnel, with the patients, their families, and visitors must demonstrate those attitudes and appreciations which she wants her staff to show toward others.

The head nurse must understand the aim of medical therapy for each patient and know what nursing care he needs. She must be capable of assessing the *nursing* needs of each patient. She must be capable of helping others to understand those needs and to plan how to meet the needs. In other words, every head nurse must be a master of her profession—a specialist not in nursing techniques but rather in the giving of nursing care.

The Relationships and Responsibilities of the Head Nurse in Team Nursing. Team nursing will work only to the degree to which the head nurse will allow it to function. The fact that she is efficient in managing her unit or that she insists upon her staff doing their work thoroughly does not presuppose that she can, or will, allow team nursing to function to its fullest extent. The head nurse who refuses to allow anyone else to assume additional responsibility or to make any decisions without consulting her is unable to delegate any of her authority and is, therefore, incapable of functioning within the framework of the principles of team nursing.

Good leadership by the head nurse is essential if team nursing is to be effectively practiced in her unit. She must believe wholeheartedly in the philosophy of the team plan and provide an example of democratic leadership, which can serve as a guide to the team leaders. Such a head nurse will give each team leader every opportunity for personal growth and self-expression, helping her to acquire a broader understanding of the meaning and practice of democratic leadership. She will give her the opportunity to develop those skills in the fields of administration, supervision, and teaching necessary for her to lead her team effectively. The fact that the head nurse delegates some of her duties and responsibilities to each of her team leaders does not mean that she loses prestige; rather, the need for her leadership, supervision and help increases as she guides her staff in the development of their skills and capabilities.

ONE OF THE MAIN RESPONSIBILITIES OF THE HEAD NURSE IS TO DELEGATE. The ability to delegate wisely is an important technique of leadership that the head nurse must develop. Even when she delegates responsibility for patient care, she still has the overall responsibility for providing effective care for every patient on her unit.

In team nursing the head nurse allows the team leader to manage and supervise her team; however, she may need to offer suggestions and help to the team leader in order to help her become more skillful in these techniques. She may also have to help some team leaders in planning nursing care for those patients who have complex problems.

OTHER RESPONSIBILITIES OF THE HEAD NURSE. Team nursing allows the head nurse more time to assume those responsibilities that are rightfully hers. She will be able to plan the work of her unit more efficiently and give her staff better supervision, including teaching and guidance, while they work. She can spend more time in evaluation of the performance of her staff as individuals and as a team and give additional advice and help as necessary.

She will also be able to spend more time with the patients, determining their needs and coordinating all hospital and community services to meet these needs. She can plan her own work so that she can attend the various conferences and meetings without worrying about her unit. In other words, she has time to be a head nurse.

The assignment of personnel to each team is an important

function of the head nurse, for she will need to consider the capabilities of each team leader as well as of the team members. She must insure that each team is composed of individuals who can work together harmoniously, each one complementing the abilities of the others. If she is not required to make time schedules, she may make suggestions to the person responsible for staffing in order to maintain a stable group whenever possible, thus providing a situation that can promote greater personal satisfaction for each team member and assure better continuity in patient care. She must also plan so that there will be no delay in the giving of team reports and no conflict in the times when the various teams hold their conferences. The head nurse will need to revise the membership of the team as some employees resign or rotate to other shifts and new people are employed. The orientation of recent employees is an important responsibility of the head nurse and must include an explanation of the philosophy of team nursing, the worker's contribution to the team, an introduction to all personnel on the unit, information about what her work will include, and how to do it, along with a tour to show her the physical layout of the unit.

Although the team leader may be given the responsibility of making the individual assignments to her team, the head nurse must designate the patients to be cared for by each group. She will need to revise the groups of patients as their conditions change or as some are discharged and others are admitted. Assigning an equal number of patients to each team is not always a fair distribution of responsibility. The head nurse must know the patients and their needs well enough so that she can determine the quantity of nursing care and the length of time needed to complete it. Although the number of team members will be determined in part by available personnel, all teams need not be the same size. If the physical layout of the ward is such that the patients are divided equally among the teams, the head nurse may need to revise the number on each team proportionate to the nursing care that must be given and the ability of team members to give that care.

Another major responsibility of the head nurse is that of teaching each team leader the principles of management and supervision, which are necessary to make her leadership more effective. The head nurse should evaluate the experience and potentialities of each staff nurse. If the person is a recent graduate or a new employee with relatively little experience, the head nurse must work closely with her, helping her to plan, supervise, and evaluate the nursing care given by her team. The person who has been away from nursing for a period of time and is now returning to active duty presents an entirely different problem. In addition to becoming acquainted with her duties and responsibilities under the team plan, this person will need to learn the new treatments and techniques that have developed with the recent changes in medicine and nursing. She may have a feeling of insecurity during this learning period and needs the assurance that the head nurse is someone to whom she can go for advice and information. The part-time employee offers still another problem, since the head nurse must try to fit this individual in where she will be most useful. Because she may be unfamiliar with the patients or with recent changes in hospital policy, the head nurse must give her additional help and supervision in order to insure the giving of safe nursing care along with deriving adequate personal satisfaction from her work.

The head nurse is the person to whom the team leader should go when she encounters problems she cannot solve. These may concern the identification of patient needs and nursing problems or the evaluation of the results of nursing care. Another type of problem may be related to the organization of team activities so that the group can do its work more easily and efficiently. Errors in patient care, either of omission or commission, must be reported to the head nurse as soon as they are recognized. She is the one who must decide what action is necessary and must notify those people who are affected. A problem of public relations involving a patient, his family, or his friends must also be referred immediately to the head nurse, since this is related to public good-will toward the hospital itself. In addition, any personnel problems are of immediate concern to the head nurse, because a problem in team relationships will often give rise to other problems. The head nurse must be willing to help the team leader arrive at an acceptable solution to her problems. On occasion, she may decide to refer the matter to the departmental supervisor for further study.

Every head nurse must be a leader. She is responsible for the patient care given by her staff to each patient; she influences their attitudes toward their work and toward the patients; she acts as an example — both as a citizen and as a nurse. She can never delegate or ignore these responsibilities.

There are times when the head nurse may have to function more specifically as a team leader. She may be the only professional nurse available, or she may need to be the leader of one of the teams. Although such situations are not ideal, the head nurse who is efficient can function in both capacities for a short time. Certainly, she should never allow the giving of nursing care to lapse into the old functional method of assgnment.

If you find yourself in this dual role, take a really critical look at all the things you think *you* have to do — checking and ordering supplies, checking charge slips, checking lab and x-ray slips, copying time sheets, recording TPR's, or whatever it is. Which is more important — the patient or the paper work? Oh, I know you cannot take care of the patient unless you have linen to change his bed; the

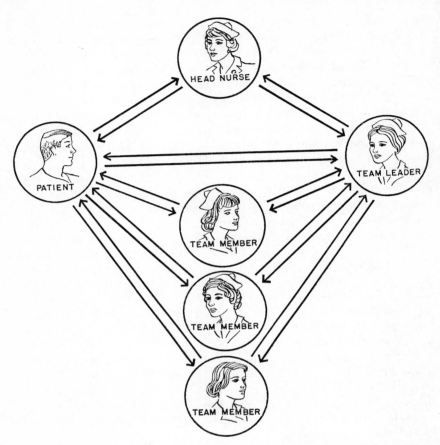

Figure 9. Effective communication never travels in one direction only.

patient will be upset if he doesn't get his lunch; the doctor will be unhappy if the laboratory work is not done; the nursing office will call if the time sheets do not reach there! But are *you* the only one who is intellectually capable of doing this paper work? Which requires more knowledge—giving Mrs. Brown the nursing care that she needs or copying words or figures from one piece of paper to another? Be honest with yourself. Is a nursing education necessary for all this paper work?

Your main concern should be that your team members are aware not only of *what* they should do but also of *how* they should do it. The direction and guidance that you give to the team as a whole and to each member as an individual is extremely important; therefore, you must keep them informed and expect them to report their observations to you.

The head nurse can also contribute directly to the work of the team in other ways. Since she has the over-all responsibility for the

nursing care given to the patients on her station, she must be interested in the nursing care plans, must help in keeping them up to
date, and must encourage the team to use them. She may wish to
attend the team conferences, where she can act as a resource person,
offering her suggestions concerning patient needs which she has
observed. She could also offer these suggestions during the patient
report.

Effective two-way communication is an essential in team nursing — within the team, between the teams, and between the team
leaders and head nurse. This should be a continuous process in
which everyone feels free and comfortable enough to offer her
observations, ideas, and suggestions for making the work of the team
more efficient and the care of the patient more effective.

RESPONSIBILITIES OF THE TEAM LEADER

In team nursing the head nurse delegates to the registered
nurse who is team leader, some of the techniques of management
and supervision related to the activities of her team. The team leader
also has the responsibility for providing the care needed by her
patients. In carrying out these functions she uses all the techniques
that have been discussed in Parts II and III.

The Team Leader Must Provide Leadership. First of all, she
must be willing to accept the responsibilities of leadership and be
able to use the various techniques that result in effective leadership.
She must be able to inspire people to want to do good work and be
able to work effectively with people. In other words, she must follow
the Decalogue for Leadership.

**The Team Leader, with the Help of the Head Nurse, Must
Cultivate Team Spirit.** Whether you are working in an area where
team nursing has been practiced for some time or are in the process
of instituting the team plan, proper preparation of all personnel is
necessary if team spirit is to develop. The spirit of cooperation
within the team necessary for effective group action, begins with
your own belief in the philosophy of team nursing and with your
attitudes toward your work and toward your team members as individuals. You must be enthusiastic about this method of planning
nursing care, for, if you are not, your own feelings of resentment
and defeat will be transmitted to your team, and you will never win
their full cooperation. You must recognize that each person has
something worthwhile to contribute to the welfare of the patient,
and, in addition, you must be able to communicate to each team
member your appreciation of her capabilities. You must have a
sincere desire to be a leader, not for the glory of the title or the
position, but for the satisfaction you obtain from working with and
helping people.

The focal point in cultivating team spirit is having a common goal — in this case, the giving of good nursing care. In all that you and your team do, this thought must be emphasized — together, the team can give better nursing care than a number of people working independently.

All members of the team must understand the principles upon which the team plan is founded and the way in which it functions. They must understand the ways of coordinating all activities of the individual members of the team to provide total nursing care for the patient. They must understand the reasons for, and the methods of using, the conference and the nursing care plan for planning and giving patient care. This information should be explained to them before team nursing is started. They should be allowed to ask questions and to discuss how the team plan would affect them and their work. Even after the team plan is instituted, this instruction should be continued, especially as new employees join the group. The team leader is the one who must reinforce this instruction by giving additional explanations, but she will generate the best enthusiasm and cooperation by her own example.

You cannot set yourself apart from your team. Telling them to work together will never be so effective as working with them yourself. Your actions must demonstrate the idea of *our* work together, rather than *your* work and *my* work.

You cannot stop at the end of the preliminary period of preparation if your group is to develop into a team, cemented together by a spirit of cooperation and a desire to achieve the common goal. Team spirit must be continually nurtured and encouraged to grow. Each person has the basic need for approval. She wants to do that which will satisfy this need, but in order to do so, she must know what she is to do and how to do it. Communication is important in any cooperative effort. Your ability to put your ideas across and to receive ideas from others is essential to the mutual understanding that must precede effective team work. You must help each person to gain a clear understanding of what she is to do and how her work is important to the patient. Show confidence in her ability to do her work, then do not forget to praise her for work well-done, or to criticize constructively and fairly when she should be better.

Not only must the individual be given recognition and help, but also the team as a whole. Emphasize that each person as a member of the team shares in the responsibility for giving good patient care, and that, when the patient is satisfied, the entire team, not one individual alone, shares in the credit.

The Team Leader Must Plan, Organize, and Direct the Activities of Her Team. She is a manager of patient care. These activities are related not only to the technical care based upon the doctor's orders but also to the nursing care based on the nursing diagnosis and nursing orders.

The team leader should make the assignments and explain them to her team. She must use the capabilities of each team member to the fullest extent. The L.P.N. must be allowed to use her knowledge and technical skills to care for those patients whose care is beyond the ability of the nursing assistant. With supervision and help the L.P.N. may be assigned to technical procedures, such as giving medications or those involving sterile technique.

The assignments that the team leader takes for herself will be determined by her personal philosophy about nursing and nursing care, by the abilities of her team members, and by hospital policy. In team nursing the team leader should do those things for the patient which others cannot do because of lack of knowledge or skill or because hospital policy forbids. In other words, she will need to give some aspects of nursing care because the team members cannot meet the specific needs of the patient. The team leader may decide to bathe and care for a critically ill patient, or perhaps work very closely with the person who is assigned to care for him. She may decide to talk with a patient who shows extreme anxiety or despair due to ordered diagnostic tests or therapy.

Personally, I do not feel that the team leader must give *all* the medications or do *all* the charting if there is someone else on the team who can assume these duties. If we allow the nurses' aide to care for critically ill patients, then she certainly is capable of putting on a sheet of paper what she did and what she saw. Rather than functioning as a ward secretary and physicians' assistant, the team leader should concern herself with her primary responsibility—the patient and his needs.

The team leader may have to use the principles of work simplification in order to arrange these activities more efficiently. She will certainly be required to establish priorities of care, determining out of the many needs and problems displayed by the patient which ones demand immediate attention from the team each day.

The Team Leader Must Supervise—That Is, Observe, Evaluate, and Teach—Her Team Members. She must remember that her coworkers have needs that should be met in order to provide job satisfaction. She must recognize when a worker is unsure of herself either in performing a nursing procedure or in being with a patient. On such occasions the team leader must give this person the help and support that she wants and needs. Her leadership must help the group realize the objective of individualized patient care. They must be able to learn from her practice the techniques of good human relationships with patients and with their families, visitors, and hospital personnel.

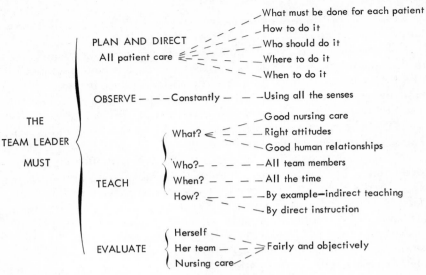

Figure 10. Activities of the team leader.

The Team Leader is Responsible for Maintaining the Nursing Care Plan. She makes the initial entries as soon as possible after the admission of the patient. She continues to add to the care plan whenever new information is available. She may determine patient needs and suggest care whenever she talks with the patients and their families, when her team members report to her, or when the doctor changes his orders. She must keep the nursing care plan up to date so that it will be of help to the nursing staff.

The Team Leader Conducts the Nursing Care Planning Conference. This is usually called the team conference. She evaluates the existing plan of care and together with her team revises and adds to it as they discuss the patient and how they can help him. On occasion she may call upon other members of the health team, e.g., the dietitian, social worker, or public health nurse, to help with specific aspects of the nursing care plan.

The Team Leader is Responsible for Maintaining Good Communication. We have already said that the team leader maintains the nursing care plan which is so important in maintaining communication among the nursing staff and insuring continuity of nursing care.

The team leader ensures that her team is kept informed. She either gives them the report or provides the opportunity for them to get it. She explains their assignments so that they know not only *what* they are to do but also *how* and *why*. As additional information comes to her during her on-duty time, she passes it on to her group. She insists that they keep her informed, telling her about their observations and problems encountered as they took care of the patients. She passes on all pertinent information to the doctor and the head nurse.

In order to increase her abilities in the field of management the team leader should be helped and encouraged to do as much supervision as she is capable of doing. We mean here, of course, that supervision which is the assistance and guidance of her team, necessary for good nursing care. Because of her close relationship with her team, the team leader has a better opportunity to give this kind of supervision than any other person who shares in this responsibility.

Am I a good team leader? *Answer each question by placing a check in the column that you believe best describes your performance.*

	1 Always	2 Often	3 Rarely
1. Do I believe that team nursing will work?			
2. Is my work a good example to others?			
3. Am I enthusiastic about my work?			
4. Do I try to learn as much as possible about every part of my job?			
5. Am I able to control my temper?			
6. Do I think before I speak?			
7. Do I admit it when I am wrong?			
8. Do I try to understand the other person's viewpoint?			
9. Do I feel that each team member is important in caring for the patient?			
10. Am I able to plan ahead?			
11. Am I systematic about doing my own work?			
12. Do I show my confidence in my team?			
13. Do I consider both the worker and the patient when I plan the assignments?			
14. Do I give a complete report to every team member?			
15. Do I ask more often than I command?			
16. Does my team voluntarily seek my advice?			
17. Do I check to determine that all assignments have been completed properly?			
18. Do I try to be objective in evaluating the work of others?			
19. Do I try to find out all the facts before I draw my conclusion?			
20. Do I offer praise often?			
21. Do I inform my team members of their progress?			
22. Do I try to help each member of my team improve?			
23. Do I encourage discussion during the team conference?			
24. Do I keep the nursing care plans up to date?			
25. Do I use the nursing care plans?			

Each check in column 1 gives you 4 points, column 2 gives you 2 points, column 3 no points. Total your score.

A score of

92 and over — Congratulations on your excellent leadership!

82 to 91 — Satisfactory, but some improvement is needed.

Below 82 — Start planning at once ways to increase your skills in leadership.

RESPONSIBILITIES OF THE TEAM MEMBERS

Team members are expected to work cooperatively with each other and with their team leader. Each person is expected to give the best care to each patient that she is capable of giving. The team as a whole must realize the contribution that each person makes to the welfare of the patient.

Each team member must be willing to contribute to the nursing care plan during the discussion at the team conference or at report by giving her observations accurately and suggesting ways of care that may help a particular patient.

While the L.P.N. cannot function as the team leader, she is a great asset to the team because of her skill in performing many of the therapeutic techniques. She may need some help from the team leader to adapt a procedure to the individual patient. Furthermore, because she has more knowledge about patient care than does the nurses' aide, she is better qualified to work with patients who need skillful care and understanding.

The nursing assistants or aides need much help and supervision, especially until they gain a great amount of experience. However, in nursing situations today they are important in helping team nursing to function effectively. Most aides are very interested in their patients and are anxious to help them as much as possible. When the team leader gives directions clearly and offers help and teaching as needed, these team members are capable of giving excellent patient care.

QUESTIONS ASKED ABOUT THE DUTIES OF
THE STAFF IN TEAM NURSING

Should there be one report only, for everyone, or should there be one report for the nurses and one for the team members? My personal belief is that it makes little difference if everyone receives one report or if the team leaders hear the report given by the previous shift, and then relay the pertinent information to their teams.

Should the head nurse or the team leader report to the oncoming shift? Whichever method is used, there must be good communication between head nurse and team leader. Since the head nurse has the over-all responsibility for everything that goes on in her unit, she must be kept fully informed by the team leaders, concerning their work and any difficulties they encounter. The head nurse, in turn, must relay all pertinent information to the team leaders if they are to function properly. The head nurse may wish to delegate to the team leader the responsibility for reporting on those patients cared for by her team; however, the head nurse must attend this report to insure its completeness by supplying additional information whenever necessary.

How can I overcome my reluctance to correct the members of my team? Perhaps part of your reluctance stems from your idea of how supervision is given. If you think of it as a means of helping your team while they are working, you may have less difficulty in showing them how to do better—whether it is because they are doing something incorrectly or because they should become more skillful in their work.

If you are a nursing student or a recent graduate and, therefore, feel reluctant because of your youth or lack of experience, I am sure that this situation will correct itself in time. Meanwhile, whenever you try to help your team members improve, indicate to them that you are using information or techniques that your clinical instructors, supervisors, or head nurses have found helpful, thereby transferring some of their authority and experience to yourself. If a situation develops that you cannot handle, you should discuss the matter with your head nurse.

Should team nursing be practiced during all three shifts or only during the day shift? Team nursing can be used throughout the entire 24 hours, with each team having a conference and planning or revising nursing care plans. If you do not yet have team nursing on all shifts, you should make sure that the nursing care plans are used around the clock.

How can a registered nurse, when she works part-time and must relieve either the team leaders or ancillary personnel, fit into the team? As a general rule, the fewer the hours worked each week, or the more widely spaced those hours are within the week, the more difficult it would be, I believe, for this nurse to assume the responsibilities of team leadership. Her unfamiliarity with the patients, their needs, and their treatment would make it almost impossible for her to give more than functional care. Furthermore, she would probably have to refer the questions asked by her team to the head nurse. This practice of referring them to someone else for advice was one point criticized often by the nurses' aides in answer to their questionnaire, and may have been the reason for their comment that they liked best the team leader "who knows her job."

If, of necessity, the part-time nurse must work as team leader, even though she is not acquainted with the patients, she must receive a thorough report and orientation to her patients from the head nurse. In addition, the head nurse will need to work more closely with her throughout the day, helping her to direct and supervise the work of her team. The head nurse may also have to assume the responsibility for conducting the team conference and checking the nursing care plans.

It would be much better if the part-time registered nurse, especially if she works only one or two days a week, could be assigned as a member of a team, relieving the team leader of some of her responsibilities, such as helping the team members care for those patients who are most ill. In this way the team leader will have more time for the supervision of the team as a whole.

How can team nursing be carried on when one team leader goes to a meeting at 1 p.m., leaving one other team leader on duty until 3 o'clock? Before the one leader leaves, she should report to the other team leader about the nursing her team has completed and what remains to be done. The two teams then become one larger team under the direction of the remaining team leader. At times, the head nurse may be the only professional nurse on duty. She then becomes the leader not only because she is head nurse and is responsible for all nursing care which her patients receive but also because as a professional nurse she must assume responsibility for directing and supervising the personnel with less knowledge than herself.

How can a team leader do her own work for the day? Whenever possible you should start your planning on the day preceding the use of the plans. You can start as soon as you know what personnel will be on your team and what patients you will be caring for. If you know these patients, you will be familiar with the care each one needs. If not, now is the time to become acquainted. Ideally, the team leader should be given the responsibility of planning the assignments for her team members; however this may be modified to meet the policies of each hospital. If you do have this responsibility, you may want to arrange the assignments also, although it is permissible to wait until you have visited each patient after hearing the patient report. In either case, you should give some preliminary thought to the duties to be done on the following day and how they can be organized. Much of the preliminary planning involves evaluating each patient and his needs and determining priorities in nursing techniques and care.

After you hear the patient report from the previous shift, you will need to visit each patient to evaluate his current condition for yourself. Your team members may be passing out bath supplies, taking temperatures, or doing other incidental duties during this time. You will not be able to spend much time with each patient; therefore, you should plan beforehand what you wish to observe and what information to obtain from the patient. Use this information, together with that obtained from the report, to adjust or make out the team assignments according to the needs of the patients and the abilities of your team members. Determine which patients need to receive their care first and how to correlate your care with that to be given by other departments within the hospital.

Your group should meet together to receive their report, or, if they attend the one given by the previous shift, you should meet together now to discuss the assignments and the methods of coordinating the activities of the team as a whole. Knowing how everyone will be working together encourages team spirit and the desire to participate.

As your team members carry out their duties, you do those things you had planned for yourself. In addition, you must circulate among your team members, helping with and directing the care they are giving. This is an important aspect in the leadership of your team. Give praise for good work, correct and teach when necessary, encourage the group to work together, be available and willing to answer questions and to help with the care of patients as necessary. If you have many duties of your own, finding the time to circulate in this way becomes a problem, yet it must be done if you are to lead your group. Perhaps you can delegate some of your other duties to another team member. Sometimes the problem is one of better work organization. Whatever the situation, you must plan to give this help as you go about your own duties.

Throughout the day, a continuous flow of communication is necessary between patient and team, including yourself; between you and your team members; and between the head nurse and yourself. Communication is a necessary ingredient of coordinated activity and effective team work.

Cooperative planning of nursing care occurs during the team conference under your guidance and direction. As a result, the nursing care plans are kept up-to-date, and necessary revisions are made when changes in the patient's progress are indicated by your own observations and by the reports of your team members.

Your team members should report to you immediately when they observe anything significant about the patient or when they encounter any problem in the care of the patient; however, you will need to teach them what is important, for they will not always realize what is significant and what is not. These reports cannot take the place of the final report each one gives before going off duty. At that time, by referring to the care plans and your own work plan, you should make certain that all aspects of nursing care and all additional duties have been completed. Record important observations on the patient's charts. Relay this information to the head nurse and to the oncoming team leaders.

Before your day is finished, you must evaluate the effectiveness of your own leadership and the nursing care given by your team. Determine how well the team worked together. Look back over the day's work for any areas that could have been improved. Finally, you must plan for tomorrow.

STUDY QUESTIONS

1. Discuss how the team leader can give a "psychological paycheck" to each of her team members.

2. Plan the individual assignments for a typical team assigned to care for an average group of patients. How are the individual needs of the patients assigned? How is this information given to the team? How did you determine the sequence of duties? How is this indicated to each team member? How are the capabilities of each team member, including the team leader, utilized?

3. List as many factors as possible that will stimulate a spirit of cooperation within the team.

4. What personal qualities in the team leader aid cooperation?

5. How much responsibility can be assumed by a team member for planning her own work?

6. What managerial functions does the team leader use during this period of preparation?

7. What specific information should be included for a recently employed practical nurse and nurses' aide on your station during orientation as given by a team leader?

8. What are the characteristics of a good patient report? What information should be included?

9. What are the characteristics of a good assignment?

10. What helpful suggestions could you give to an individual who is having difficulty in organizing her work?

11. Give the various reasons why some people are unable to complete their assignments on time.

12. Write a job description for a team leader including the personal qualifications and duties and responsibilities.

13. Rewrite the job descriptions for each of the following and indicate the person's responsibilities in team nursing:
   a. For a head nurse
   b. For a licensed practical nurse
   c. For a nursing assistant

14. List as many specific duties as you can that are now performed by the head nurse. Analyze each one. Which ones could be performed by someone else? Why? Which ones must remain the responsibility of the head nurse? Why?

15. Make specific suggestions as to how the head nurse can participate in team activities.

16. List specific duties now being performed by the team leader. Analyze each one. Which ones could be performed by someone else? Why? Which ones should she be doing that she is not now performing?

Chapter 12

The Team and Other
Hospital Personnel

Many people in the hospital, while not a part of any team, may be affected by team activities. When the team method is initiated, all hospital personnel must acquire a working knowledge about how it functions and how its activities will affect the responsibilities they may have for the patient.

UNIT MANAGER AND WARD SECRETARY
AND TEAM NURSING

These people may have various titles but they are always concerned with administrative activities in the patient unit. The ward or unit manager serves as a liaison between the nursing staff on the station and other departments. He also answers the telephone, and arranges for repairs, extra supplies, dietary trays, and other necessities. Either the manager or secretary is responsible for the transfer of doctor's orders, arranging for laboratory and x-ray examinations, requisitioning drugs and dressings, and sending in charges for supplies as they are used.

When the head nurse is relieved of these time-consuming duties, she has time to interview patients, teach and help the team leaders, coordinate the care given by her entire staff, and assist in the planning of nursing care.

One of the problems occurring between the manager and the secretary and the team is poor communication. The manager must relay information promptly and accurately to and from team leaders, to and from doctors, to and from various hospital departments. With experience and a desire to make the system work, the manager, head nurse, and team leaders can set up general guides so that information will move effectively from the source to the person who needs it.

Another problem which may occur involves interpersonal relationships among the nursing staff and the unit administrative people, especially when the team leaders work closely with the manager. Job descriptions for the unit manager and the ward secretary must define the specific limits of their duties and responsibilities. Similar information should be given for the positions of head nurse and team leader. There must be no overlapping. Every responsibility must be clearly indicated. When people know what their job includes and how their activities are related to those of other personnel, cooperation and harmonious working relationships are more likely to be present.

Habits are hard to break. For many years the head nurse has traditionally performed her work behind the desk in the nursing station. When the unit manager takes over this geographic location and some of the duties the head nurse has always thought to be part of her job, she tends to feel lost. She may find it hard to divorce herself from these activities as long as the title of head nurse remains. Some hospitals find that she is able to make the change more easily when her title is changed, for example, to nursing care coordinator, and an entirely new job description is made up for her.[*]

THE NURSING SUPERVISOR AND TEAM NURSING

The role of the nursing supervisor has been much discussed in professional circles, with the result that there seems to be a question concerning just what her role should be. Since the supervisor is usually concerned with an entire department, made up of several nursing units, she has the opportunity to get a broader picture of how the nursing needs of the patients are being met, how the various members of her department are working together, and how her department can work more cooperatively with the other departments in the hospital. Because of her additional skills and experience, she should be able to help the head nurses in solving the problems arising on the various stations. She can also help in estab-

---

*Hass, Ruth L.: "Our Nurses Are Nursing." *Minnesota Nursing Accent.* Minnesota Nurses' Ass'n. June, 1968, p. 79.

lishing and keeping open the lines of communication between hospital administration and the head nurses.

She can also play an important part in the functioning of team nursing, first, by helping the head nurses to develop a better understanding of the team members' place in the team plan and, secondly, by helping them to become more democratic in their leadership. The nursing supervisor must demonstrate her interest in the effective functioning of the team members. She is in an excellent position to interpret the aims of the team plan to hospital administration and to explain how it can be made to work more efficiently.

Perhaps one of her biggest opportunities for increasing the scope of her supervision is in the field of research. Whenever nursing service problems are referred to her, she should try to plan cooperatively with the personnel involved so that a better method of giving nursing care may be discovered through the solution of these problems. She should always be on the lookout for more efficient work methods, either by revising established procedures or by using different equipment.

THE CLINICAL SPECIALIST AND TEAM NURSING

Some nurses are currently trying to define their roles as clinical specialists. Rinehart implies that the head nurse at the present time may fill this role because she manages patient care, i.e., plans, organizes, directs, and controls that care.*

In some situations a nurse with special preparation in a clinical area may be given the job title of clinical specialist. In this more specific classification the nurse is directly concerned with the management of nursing care of those patients assigned to her. She is not a part of the staff on any one unit but is responsible for her patients wherever they may be located. She is free to visit them several times during the day or night and may interview them on admission, make a nursing diagnosis and give nursing orders, which she passes on to the nursing staff who will carry them out, or give her patients nursing care herself if she decides it is necessary.

She is not the team leader according to the definition of this position in team nursing; however, she can function effectively as a source of information to help the team determine what the problems of their patients are and how they can give them the most help. She can increase their understanding and acceptance of the patient and

---

*Rinehart, Elma L.: *Management of Nursing Care.* Macmillan Co., 1969, p. 39.

his needs. She should be an ex-officio member of the team confer-ence whenever the care of one of her patients is being discussed.

The degree to which she can encourage the team to give better patient care is limited only by her knowledge of behavioral, medical, and nursing principles and her ability to establish good working relationships with the nursing staff.

THE NURSING STUDENT AND TEAM NURSING

Team nursing can be either an asset or a liability to the educa-tion of the nursing student, depending upon the interest and skill of the head nurse and the team leader in teaching the techniques of good nursing care and in giving democratic leadership. Nursing service personnel are so often concerned with the care of patients today that they forget about the person who will be giving nursing care tomorrow, or next year, or two years from now. The kind of care the patients will receive in the future can be only as good as the care the nursing student learns to give today. However, it is no longer sufficient for her to know what good nursing care is and how to give it herself; she must be given the opportunity to learn and to practice those skills needed in directing and supervising others in the giving of total patient care. She must recognize the importance of good human relations and learn to work cooperatively with others in meeting the nursing care needs of the patients.

Early Experience in Team Nursing. The nursing student should spend some time as a team member during the early part of her clinical experience; in this way, she can learn through observa-tion and personal experience how the team functions. She can see teamwork in action and learn the importance of cooperation in the giving of good patient care. As she attends the team conferences, she can learn how patient-centered care is planned, and as she receives a report and listens to the explanation of the individual assignments to the team members, she will realize how that plan is carried out.

School policies must be followed when planning the student's assignment; however, it may be made out by the head nurse or the team leader in cooperation with the clinical instructor. Every assign-ment must be planned on the basis of the learning needs of the student. Early in her experience she needs to gain skill in the perfor-mance of nursing techniques and in the actual planning, giving, and evaluating of the patient's care. As she carries out this assignment, the team leader should be willing to offer assistance whenever the student shows a need. Although the student is concerned with giving complete care to some patients, she must also be made to feel that she is a part of the team, perhaps by being assigned to assist with certain parts of a patient's care which an aide cannot perform. Thus, the student begins to learn how to work with people and how to coordinate the work of several persons to provide individualized patient care.

Since the team leader is responsible for the nursing care given by her team, she will want to supervise and help the student in the giving of that care. However, she shares this responsibility with the head nurse and the clinical instructor, for all three must work together to plan a good learning experience for the student and to help her gain the necessary knowledge, understanding, and skills required by the professional nurse.

The Nursing Student as Team Leader. As the nursing student becomes more skillful in performing the required techniques, in understanding the needs of her patients, and in helping them to solve their problems, she should learn how to guide and direct others in giving patient-centered care. This may be done by giving her the opportunity to act as team leader.

If the student is to acquire acceptable attitudes toward and appreciations of her professional responsibilities as a leader, her experience as a team leader must be carefully planned and closely supervised. She must recognize the importance of human relations and learn to apply the principles of democratic leadership in all her team relations. She must be helped and encouraged to increase her skills in planning and evaluating patient-centered care, in solving nursing problems, and in directing and supervising the work of others. She must learn what team leadership requires and how to effectively meet her responsibilities toward her patients, the members of her team, and herself.

Throughout the entire clinical experience of the nursing student, emphasis must be placed on methods of individualizing the nursing care of each patient. The head nurse and the team leader must be especially careful to plan her assignments in such a way that the idea of performing nursing techniques on a functional basis is minimized and, instead, the part each has in the total care of the patient is emphasized. Especially when acting as team leader, the nursing student must be made to realize that her responsibility to her team and to her patients goes beyond the mere giving of treatments and medications and doing the necessary recording on the patient's chart. However, if she is to realize and appreciate fully the scope of this responsibility, she must have been brought up in an atmosphere of teamwork from the very beginning of her clinical experience and have had the opportunity to observe other team leaders as they effectively put into practice the principles of team leadership.

THE CLINICAL INSTRUCTOR AND TEAM NURSING

Cooperation between the team leader, head nurse, and clinical instructor is absolutely essential in order to provide the nursing student with a good learning experience and adequate supervision. Each one has an important contribution to make to the education of the student, but, if an atmosphere conducive to learning is to be provided, each must understand the aims and problems of the others. It is important that both the head nurse and the team leader remember that the nursing student is present on the ward primarily for the purpose of learning and only secondarily for service. Until they gain an appreciation of this fact, the nursing student will fail to gain a complete experience either in the giving of nursing care or in an appreciation of her responsibilities as a professional nurse. Every nursing student must be provided with a good clinical education if the head nurse is to have, in the future, well-prepared nurses who will be able to give good nursing care and to assume the responsibilities required of them. The student's attitudes about what her role in nursing is, and how to fulfill it, are being formed by her experiences today.

The clinical instructor should strive to interpret the aims of nursing education to the head nurse and team leader and to help them in planning the student's experience so that these aims can be met. On the other hand, the clinical instructor must realize that the immediate care of the patient is of primary concern to the nursing service personnel; therefore, she must be willing to work with these people in supervising and guiding the student.

Especially in planning the assignment for the nursing student, the clinical instructor, the head nurse, and the team leader must work closely together. The activities of the station will become disorganized unless this assignment is planned well and all three know exactly what the student is to do. More important, the patient and part of his care may be neglected unless all are kept informed. However, the head nurse and team leader must remember that occasionally a student's assignment may need to be changed on short notice in order to provide her with experience in an unforeseen learning situation which arises. On the other hand, the clinical instructor should try to look ahead so that such changes are made with a minimum amount of confusion.

The clinical instructor should be an ex-officio member of any team of which the student is a member, especially if the student is acting as team leader. She will need to work with the student in identifying the needs of the patients and in planning their care. She will also need to help her to acquire the necessary skills to effectively lead the team conference, to supervise her team in giving the patient care as indicated on the care plan, and finally, in evaluating the effectiveness of that care and of her own leadership.

PERSONNEL FROM VARIOUS DEPARTMENTS AND TEAM NURSING

Persons from almost every hospital department will at one time or another have to work with members of the team; consequently, they should have a basic working knowledge of the mechanics of team nursing.

Dietary workers may report to the team leader that between-meal nourishments are delivered. The dietitian may be asked to explain to the team what she is teaching the patient about his diet so they can reinforce her explanations.

The physiotherapist can help the team learn what they can do for their patient to keep him from losing ground over the weekend when the department is closed. The team leader may pass on to the x-ray technician information that she has found helpful so that the same approach can be used by the technician to gain the patient's cooperation during his examination or therapy.

The team plan can be constantly expanded as the personnel realize to a greater extent what can be accomplished through team-work and make use of every opportunity for personal growth. Continuous in-service programs for the professional nurses must be carried on to help them increase their understanding of team nurs-ing and ways of applying its principles to their own situation. The training of the nonprofessional personnel cannot be carried on sole-ly by the head nurse and the team leader. A program of instruc-tion is necessary for these people, especially for those recently employed, although the head nurse and team leader will both need to reinforce and enlarge upon the teaching given in this program.

The fullest expression of the principles of team nursing will not be achieved in one month, one year, or even two years, for, as the team members gain more knowledge and understanding, so will also their concept of the work of the nursing team continue to grow. Yet team leadership will always remain a challenge to the professional nurse, and her democratic leadership will always be the key to a successful nursing team.

STUDY QUESTIONS

1. If you are associated with a school of nursing, what are its objectives? What are the means used to achieve these aims and objectives? What are the

objectives of the nursing service department? Discuss the relationships between the objectives of these two departments.

2. How could cooperation be increased between two or more departments in your hospital?

3. Discuss the responsibilities of the head nurse in your hospital for aiding in the education of the nursing student.

4. Discuss the areas in which the team leader may help in the education of the nursing student.

5. Make a job description for a unit manager and for a ward clerk or secretary. Be sure to indicate relationships between that person and the team leader and head nurse. How can you encourage good cooperation between the manager and the nursing staff? What measures could be used to aid in good communication?

6. Give specific suggestions as to how a clinical specialist can participate in team activities.

7. Discuss the role of clinical supervisor in nursing activities and in team nursing.

8. Give specific suggestions as to how the supervisor can participate in team activities.

9. Do you believe that the concept of the team plan can ever be practiced to its fullest extent? Give your reasons.

PART FOUR BIBLIOGRAPHY

Books

Peterson, Grace: *Working with Others for Patient Care.* Wm. C. Brown Company, Dubuque, Iowa, 1968.
Lambertsen, Eleanor: *Nursing Team—Organization and Functioning.* Published for the Division of Nursing Education, Bureau of Publications, Teacher's College, Columbia University, New York, 1953.
Newcomb, Dorothy Perkins: *The Team Plan, A Manual for Nursing Service Administrators.* G. P. Putnam's Sons, Inc., New York, 1953.

Pamphlets and Journals

Christman, Luther: *The Nurse Clinical Specialist.* Hospital Progress, 49:8:14, Aug., 1968.
Coletti, Angela C.: *The Head Nurse Is a Manager.* Hospital Progress, 41:3:100, March, 1960.
Cook, Billie Jo McCullars, and Festog, Eleanor I: *Talk About Team Nursing.* Am. J. Nursing, 63:11:93, Nov., 1963.
Corona, Dorothy F., and Black, Eunice E.: *One Hospital's Approach to Team Nursing.* Nurs. Outlook, 11:7:506, July, 1963.
Egolf, Marion G.: *Unit Management Program Provides More Effective Use of Personnel.* Hospitals, 43:14:77, July 16, 1969.
Elizabeth, Sister Regina: *Team Nursing Revised.* Hospital Progress, 45:7:112, July, 1964.
Fogt, Joan: *Team Nursing: Concepts and Procedures.* Hospital Progress, 45:2:65, Feb., 1964.
Fogt, Joan: *Team Nursing: Inservice Education for the Team Leader.* Hospital Progress, 45:4:31, April, 1964.
Fogt, Joan: *Team Nursing: The Team Leader.* Hospital Progress, 45:3:104, March, 1964.
Ginsberg, Frances: *How to Motivate People to Accept Change.* Modern Hospital, 111:5:114, Nov., 1968.

Gordon, Marjory: *The Clinical Specialist as Change Agent.* Nurs. Outlook, *17*:3:37, March, 1969.

Hannan, C. Phillip: *Planning and Implementing a Workable Unit Management System.* Hospital Progress, May, 1969, page 120.

Hass, Ruth L.: *Our Nurses Are Nursing.* Minnesota Nursing Agent, Minnesota Nurses' Association, June, 1968, page 79.

Johnson, Dorothy E., et al.: *The Clinical Specialist as a Practitioner.* Am. J. Nursing, *67*:11:2298, Nov., 1967.

Melody, Mary, and Clark, Genevieve: *Walking-Planning Rounds.* Am. J. Nursing, *67*:4:771, April, 1967.

Merton, Robert K.: *Relations Between Registered Nurses and Licensed Practical Nurses.* Am. J. Nursing, *62*:10:70, Oct., 1962.

Miller, Mary Annice: *Essentials for Self and Staff Improvement.* Am. J. Nursing, *61*:11:85, Nov., 1961.

Muller, Theresa G.: *The Head Nurse as a Teacher.* Nurs. Outlook, *11*:1:46, Jan., 1963.

Shepardson, Jeanette: *Developing a Job Description.* Am. J. Nursing, *62*:4:62, April, 1962.

Smith, Dorothy M.: *The Nursing Team: Fact or Fancy.* Minnesota Nursing Accent, Minnesota Nurses' Association, *36*:2:26, Feb., 1964.

Stevenson, Neva M.: *The Better Utilization of Licensed Practical Nurses.* Nurs. Outlook, *13*:7:340, July, 1965.

Williams, Margaret Aasterud: *The Myths and Assumptions About Team Nursing.* Nursing Forum, *3*:4:61, 1964.

Wood, M. Marian: *From General Duty Nurse to Team Leader.* Am. J. Nursing, *63*:1:104, Jan., 1963.

INDEX